Clinical Problem Solving in Dentistry

For Churchill Livingstone:

Commissioning Editor: Michael Parkinson
Project Development Manager: Janice Urquhart
Project Manager: Frances Affleck
Design direction: Erik Bigland
Illustrated by: Robert Britton

Clinical Problem Solving in Dentistry

EDITED BY

Edward W. Odell

Senior Lecturer and Honorary Consultant in Oral Pathology,
Guy's, King's and St Thomas' Dental Institute,
Guy's Hospital and King's College, London, UK

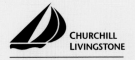

CHURCHILL
LIVINGSTONE

EDINBURGH LONDON NEW YORK PHILADELPHIA ST LOUIS
SYDNEY TORONTO 2000

CHURCHILL LIVINGSTONE
An imprint of Harcourt Publishers Limited

First published 2000
Reprinted 2000

ISBN 0 443 05631 5

British Library Cataloguing in Publication Data
A catalogue record for this book is available from the British
Library.

Library of Congress Cataloging in Publication Data
A catalog record for this book is available from the Library of
Congress.

Medical knowledge is constantly changing. As new information
becomes available, changes in treatment, procedures, equipment
and the use of drugs become necessary. The editor, contributors
and the publishers have, as far as it is possible, taken care to
ensure that the information given in this text is accurate and up to
date. However, readers are strongly advised to confirm that the
information, especially with regard to drug usage, complies with
current legislation and standards of practice.

The
publisher's
policy is to use
**paper manufactured
from sustainable forests**

Printed in China

Preface

Textbooks of clinical cases and problems have proved very popular in undergraduate and postgraduate medicine. However, they have not been developed as extensively in dentistry. This is surprising when one considers that problem solving is a basic skill for dentists, both in diagnosis as well as in the more mechanical aspects of dental treatment.

It is impossible to learn the skill of problem solving from a textbook. Rather, the purpose of this book is to help students reorganize factual knowledge in their minds. Most traditional textbooks provide information in a framework based on body systems, diseases, specialties or treatments. Knowledge structured in this way is not readily applied to clinical situations and students must mentally reorganize it, identifying common themes and links between different areas and constructing a knowledge matrix which can be more readily recalled and applied. A problem-centred approach shows students what they need to achieve.

A problem-based approach also gives the opportunity to pose the types of very practical questions which often occur in BDS or MFDS examinations but are rarely addressed directly in textbooks. I have also included some of the fundamental but perceptive questions which tend to be asked by students with little knowledge or experience.

In a traditional learning environment, many of the approaches, topics and tips explained in this book are taught in clinics. However, clinical teaching in some subjects is in danger of being compromised by reduced numbers of patients and the changing caseload in dental schools. In future, I hope that students will be able to learn some of the practicalities of patient care from books such as this, so that the limited time available in clinics can be used to maximum advantage.

I would like to thank all the authors who have contributed text and pictures to this book, many having provided input to problems other than those for which they are individually credited. My thanks are also due to Dr P. R. Morgan for reading the manuscript, and to my family, whose time I have taken to write my own contribution.

E. W. O.   London, 1999

Contributors

David W. Bartlett
Senior Lecturer in Conservative Dentistry, Guy's, King's and St Thomas' Dental Institute, Guy's Hospital and King's College, London, UK

Shahid I. Chaudhry
Honorary Clinical Assistant in Oral Medicine, Guy's, King's and St Thomas' Dental Institute, Guy's Hospital and King's College, London, UK

David C. Craig
Associate Specialist in Dental Sedation, Guy's and St Thomas' Hospital Trust, London, UK

Nicholas M. Goodger
Lecturer in Oral and Maxillofacial Surgery, Guy's, King's and St Thomas' Dental Institute, Guy's Hospital and King's College, London, UK

Mike G. Harrison
Research Fellow in Paediatric Dentistry, Guy's, King's and St Thomas' Dental Institute, Guy's Hospital and King's College; Lecturer and Honorary Consultant in Paediatric Dentistry, Eastman Dental Institute, London, UK

Peter Longhurst
Senior Lecturer and Honorary Consultant in Paediatric Dentistry, Guy's, King's and St Thomas' Dental Institute, Guy's Hospital and King's College, London, UK

Robert M. Mordecai
Senior Lecturer and Honorary Consultant in Orthodontics, Guy's, King's and St Thomas' Dental Institute, Guy's Hospital and King's College, London, UK

Edward W. Odell
Senior Lecturer and Honorary Consultant in Oral Pathology, Guy's, King's and St Thomas' Dental Institute, Guy's Hospital and King's College, London, UK

Guy D. Palmer
Senior Demonstrator in Sedation and Special Care Dentistry, Guy's, King's and St Thomas' Dental Institute, Guy's Hospital and King's College, London, UK

Richard M. Palmer
Professor of Implant Dentistry and Periodontology, Guy's, King's and St Thomas' Dental Institute, Guy's Hospital and King's College, London, UK

David R. Radford
Senior Lecturer and Honorary Consultant, Division of Prosthetic Dentistry, Guy's, King's and St Thomas' Dental Institute, Guy's Hospital and King's College, London, UK

Tara F. Renton
Senior Research Fellow and Honorary Associate Specialist in Oral and Maxillofacial Surgery, Guy's, King's and St Thomas' Dental Institute, Guy's Hospital and King's College, London, UK

David N. Ricketts
Former Lecturer in Conservative Dentistry, Guy's, King's and St Thomas' Dental Institute, Guy's Hospital and King's College, London, UK

Paul D. Robinson
Senior Lecturer and Honorary Consultant in Oral and Maxillofacial Surgery, Guy's, King's and St Thomas' Dental Institute, Guy's Hospital and King's College, London, UK

Martyn Sherriff
Senior Lecturer in Biomaterials Science, Guy's, King's and St Thomas' Dental Institute, Guy's Hospital and King's College, London, UK

Penelope J. Shirlaw
Associate Specialist in Oral Medicine, Guy's and St Thomas' Hospital Trust, London, UK

Meg Skelly
Senior Lecturer and Honorary Consultant in Dental Sedation, Guy's, King's and St Thomas' Dental Institute, Guy's Hospital and King's College, London, UK

Anwar R. Tappuni
Clinical Research Fellow in Oral Medicine, Guy's, King's and St Thomas' Dental Institute, Guy's Hospital and King's College, London, UK

Wanninayaka M. Tilakaratne
Senior Lecturer and Consultant in Oral Pathology, University of Peradeniya, Sri Lanka

Michael J. Twitchen
General Dental Practitioner, West Sussex, UK

Eric Whaites
Senior Lecturer and Honorary Consultant in Dental Radiography, Guy's, King's and St Thomas' Dental Institute, Guy's Hospital and King's College, London, UK

Contents

CASE 1

A high caries rate

Summary

A 17-year-old sixth-form college student presents at your general dental surgery with several carious lesions, one of which is very large. How should you stabilize his condition?

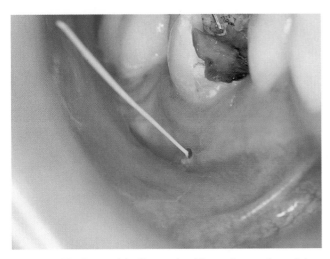

Fig. 1.1 The lower right first molar. The gutta percha point indicates a sinus opening.

HISTORY

Complaint

He complains that a filling has fallen out of a tooth on the lower right side and has left a sharp edge which irritates his tongue. He is otherwise asymptomatic.

History of complaint

The filling was placed about a year ago at a casual visit to the dentist precipitated by acute toothache triggered by hot and cold food and drink. He did not return to complete a course of treatment. He lost contact when he moved house and is not registered with a dental practitioner.

Medical history

The patient is otherwise fit and well.

EXAMINATION

Extraoral examination

He is a fit and healthy-looking adolescent. No submental, submandibular or other cervical lymph nodes are palpable and the temporomandibular joints appear normal.

Intraoral examination

The lower right quadrant is shown in Figure 1.1. The oral mucosa is healthy and the oral hygiene is reasonable. There is gingivitis in areas but no calculus is visible and probing depths are 3 mm or less. The mandibular right first molar is grossly carious and a sinus is discharging buccally. There are no other restorations in any teeth. No teeth have been extracted and the third molars are not visible. A small cavity is present on the occlusal surface of the mandibular right second molar.

■ *What further examination would you carry out?*

Tests of tooth vitality of the teeth in the region of the sinus. Even though the first molar is the most likely cause, the adjacent teeth should be tested because more than one tooth might be non-vital. The results should be compared with those of the teeth on the opposite side. Both hot/cold methods and electric pulp testing could be used because extensive reactionary dentine may moderate the response.

The first molar fails to respond to any test. All other teeth appear vital.

INVESTIGATIONS

■ *What radiographs would you take? Explain why each view is required.*

Radiograph	Reason taken
Bitewing radiographs	Primarily to detect approximal surface caries, and in this case also required to detect occlusal caries.
Periapical radiograph of the lower right first molar tooth, preferably taken with a paralleling technique	Preoperative assessment for endodontic treatment or for extraction should it be necessary.
Panoramic tomograph	Might be useful as a general survey view in a new patient and to determine the presence and position of third molars.

■ *What problems are inherent in the diagnosis of caries in this patient?*

Occlusal lesions are now the predominant form of caries in adolescents following the reduction in caries incidence over the past decades. Occlusal caries may go undetected on visual examination for two reasons. First, it starts on the

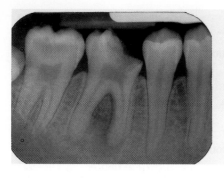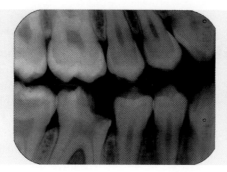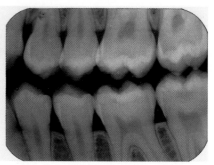

Fig. 1.2 Periapical and bitewing films.

fissure walls and is obscured by sound superficial enamel, and secondly lesions cavitate late, if at all, probably because fluoride strengthens the overlying enamel. Superimposition of sound enamel also masks small and medium-sized lesions on bitewing radiographs. The small occlusal cavity in the second molar arouses suspicion that other pits and fissures in the molars will be carious. Unless lesions are very large, extending into the middle third of dentine, they may not be detected on bitewing radiographs.

■ *The radiographs are shown in Figure 1.2. What do you see?*

The periapical radiograph shows the carious lesion in the crown of the lower right first molar to be extensive, involving the pulp cavity. The mesial contact has been completely destroyed and the molar has drifted mesially and tilted. There are periapical radiolucencies at the apices of both roots, that on the mesial root being larger. The radiolucencies are in continuity with the periodontal ligament and there is loss of most of the lamina dura in the bifurcation and around the apices.

The bitewing radiographs confirm the carious exposure and in addition reveal occlusal caries in all the maxillary and mandibular molars with the exception of the upper right first molar. No approximal caries is present.

■ *If two or more teeth were possible causes of the sinus, how might you decide which was the cause?*

A gutta percha point could be inserted into the sinus prior to taking the radiograph, as shown in Figure 1.1. A medium- or fine-sized point is flexible but resilient enough to pass along the sinus tract if twisted slightly on insertion. Points are radiopaque and can be seen on a radiograph extending to the source of the infection, as shown in another case in Figure 1.3.

DIAGNOSIS

■ *What is your diagnosis?*

The patient has a nonvital lower first molar with a periapical abscess. In addition he has a very high caries rate in a previously almost caries-free dentition.

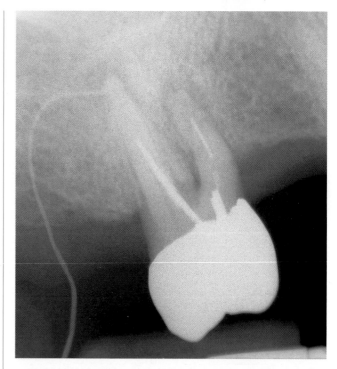

Fig. 1.3 Another case, showing gutta percha point tracing the path of a sinus.

TREATMENT

The patient is horrified to discover that his dentition is in such a poor state, having experienced only one episode of toothache in the past. He is keen to do all that can be done to save all teeth and a decision is made to try to restore the lower molar.

■ *How will you prioritize treatment for this patient? Why should treatment be provided in this sequence?*

See Table 1.1.

■ *What temporary restoration materials are available? What are their properties and in what situations are they useful?*

See Table 1.2.

Table 1.1 Sequence of treatment

Phase of treatment	Items of treatment	Reasons
Immediate phase	Caries removal from the lower right first molar, access cavity preparation for endodontics, drainage, irrigation with sodium hypochlorite and placement of a temporary restoration	Essential if the tooth is to be saved and to remove the source of the apical infection. There is also an urgent need to minimize further destruction of this tooth which may soon be unrestorable. The temporary restoration is necessary to facilitate rubber dam isolation during future endodontic treatment, and it will also stabilize the occlusion and stop mesial drift.
Stabilization of caries	Removal of caries and placement of temporary restorations in all carious teeth in visits by quadrants/two quadrants	To prevent further tooth destruction and progression to carious exposure while other phases of treatment are being carried out.
Preventive treatment	Dietary analysis, oral hygiene instruction, fluoride advice	Should start immediately and extend throughout the treatment plan, to reduce the high caries rate and ensure the long-term future of the dentition.
Permanent restoration	Will depend on what is found while placing temporary restorations	Permanent restorations may be left until last; stabilization takes priority.

Table 1.2 Temporary restoration materials

Material	Examples	Properties	Situations
Zinc oxide and eugenol pastes	Kalzinol	Bactericidal, easy to mix and place, cheap but not very strong. Easily removed.	Suitable for temporary restoration of most cavities provided there is no significant occlusal load. Endodontic access cavities.
Self-setting zinc oxide cements	Cavit Coltosol	Harden in contact with saliva. Reasonable strength and easily removed	Endodontic access cavities. No occlusal load.
Polycarboxylate cements	Poly-F	Adhesive to enamel and dentine, hard and durable.	Used when mechanical retention is poor. Strong enough to enable rubber dam placement when used in a badly broken down tooth.
Glass ionomer including silver reinforced preparations	Chem-fil Shofu Hi-Fi Ketac Silver	Adhesive to enamel and dentine, hard and durable. Good appearance.	As polycarboxylate cements and also useful in anterior teeth.

■ *Why is one molar so much more broken down than the others?*

It is difficult to be certain but the extensive caries is probably, in part, a result of the previous restoration. In view of the pattern of caries in the other molars, it seems likely that this was a large occlusal restoration and the history suggests it was placed in a vital tooth. It probably undermined the mesial cusps or marginal ridge. Three factors could have contributed to the extensive caries present only 1 year later: marginal leakage, undermining of the marginal ridge or mesial cusps leading to collapse, or failure to remove all the carious tissue from the tooth. Failure to remove all carious enamel and dentine before placing a restoration is a common cause of failure.

■ *How would you ensure removal of all carious tissue when restoring the vital molars?*

Removal of all softened carious tissue at the amelodentinal junction is essential and only stained but hard dentine can be left in place.

Removal of carious dentine over the pulp is treated differently. In a young patient with large pulp chambers there is always a tendency for the operator to be conservative but this might be counterproductive if softened or infected dentine were left below the restoration. Very soft or flaky dentine must always be removed. Slightly soft dentine can be left in situ provided a good well-sealed restoration is placed over it. Deciding whether to leave the last layers of softened dentine can be difficult and the decision rests to a degree on clinical experience. Pain associated with pulpitis indicates a need to remove more dentine or, if severe, a need for elective endodontics. Interpreting softened dentine in rapidly advancing lesions is difficult. The deepest layers are soft through demineralization but are not necessarily infected and may sometimes be left over the pulp. Also, bacterial penetration of the dentine is not reliably indicated by staining in rapidly advancing lesions. Removal of the last layers of carious dentine may require some courage in deep lesions.

Caries indicator dyes have been felt helpful in such circumstances. The dye stains the denatured collagen and matrix of dentine. However, caries detectors stain uninfected dentine which does not need to be removed and their use carries a risk of overdestructive cavity preparation.

■ What is the most important preventive procedure for this patient? Explain why.

Diet analysis. Caries requires dietary sugars, in particular sucrose, glucose and fructose, an acidogenic plaque flora and a susceptible tooth surface. Denying the plaque flora its substrate sugar is the most effective measure to halt the progression of existing lesions and prevent new ones forming. No preventive measure affecting the flora or tooth is as effective. A further advantage of emphasis on diet is that it forces the patient to acknowledge that they must take responsibility for preventing their own disease.

■ How would you evaluate a patient's diet?

Dietary analysis consists of two elements: enquiry into lifestyle and into the dietary components themselves. Information about the diet itself is of little value unless it is taken in context with the patient's lifestyle. Only dietary recommendations tailored to the patient's lifestyle are likely to be adopted.

The diet record should include all the foods and drinks consumed, the amount (in readily estimated units) and the time of eating or drinking.

In this case it should be noted that the patient is a 17-year-old student. Lifestyle often changes dramatically between the ages of 16 and 20. He may no longer be living at home and may be enjoying physical, financial and dietary independence from his parents. He may be poor and be eating a cheap carbohydrate-rich diet of snacks instead of regular meals. Long hours of studying may be accompanied by the frequent consumption of sweetened drinks.

Analysis of the diet itself may be performed in a variety of ways. The patient can be asked to recall all foods consumed over the previous 24 hours. This is not very effective, relying as it does on a good memory and honesty, and is unlikely to give a representative account. Relying on memory for more than 24 hours is too inaccurate.

The most effective method is for the patient to keep a written record of their diet for four consecutive days, including two working and two leisure days. The need for the patient to comply fully and assess their diet honestly must be stressed and, of course, the diet should not be changed because it is being recorded. Ideally the analysis should be performed before any dietary advice is given. Even the patient who does not keep an honest account has been made more aware of their diet. If they know what foods to omit from the sheet to make their dentist happy, at least the first step in an educative process has been made.

■ How will you analyse this patient's 4-day diet sheet shown in Figure 1.4? What is the cause of his caries susceptibility?

Highlight sugar-rich foods and drinks as in Figure 1.4. Note whether they are confined to meal times or whether they are **eaten frequently** and spaced throughout the day as snacks. The number of **sugar attacks should be counted** and

discussed with the patient. Also note the **consistency** of the food because dry and sticky foods take longer to be cleared from the mouth. Sugared drinks taken immediately before bed are highly significant because salivary flow is reduced during sleep and clearance time is greater. Identify foods with a high **hidden sugar** content because patients often do not realize that such foods are significant; examples are baked beans, breakfast cereals, tomato ketchup and 'plain' biscuits.

The diet sheet shows that the main problem for this patient is too many sugar-containing drinks and carbonated drinks, and frequent snacks of cake and biscuits. Most meals or snacks contain a high sugar item and some more than one. The other typical cause of a high caries rate in this age group is sweets, especially mints.

■ What advice will you give the patient?

The principles of a safer diet are shown in Table 1.3 (p. 6).

Dietary advice is almost always provided using the health-belief model of health education. However, it is well-known that education about the risks and consequences of lifestyle, habits and diet is often ineffective. It is important to judge the patient's likely compliance and provide dietary advice which can be used to make small but significant changes rather than attempting to eradicate all sugar from the diet. As the diet improves, the advice can be adapted and extended. Advice must be acceptable, practical and affordable. In this case the patient has already suffered serious consequences from his poor diet and this may help change behaviour.

The patient must be made aware that damage to teeth continues for up to 1 hour after a sugar intake. The explanation given to some patients may be no more than this simple statement. Many other patients can comprehend the concept (if not the detail) of a Stephan curve without difficulty.

The patient should be advised to use a fluoride-containing toothpaste. During the period of dietary change it would also be beneficial to use a weekly fluoride rinse as well. This could be continued for as long as the diet is felt to be unsafe.

Oral hygiene instruction is also important, but may be emphasized in a later phase of treatment. It will not stop caries progression, which is critical for this patient, and there is only a mild gingivitis.

■ Assuming good compliance and motivation, how will you restore the teeth permanently?

The mandibular right first molar requires orthograde endodontic treatment and replacement of the temporary restoration with a core. Retention for the core can be provided by residual tooth tissue, provided carious destruction is not gross. The restorative material may be packed into the pulp chamber and the first 2–3 mm of the root canal. If insufficient natural crown remains, it may be supplemented with a preformed post in the distal canals. The distal canal is not ideal, being further from the most extensively destroyed area, but it is larger.

The other molar teeth will need to have their temporary restorations replaced by definitive restorations. Caries involved only the occlusal surface but removal of these large lesions has probably left little more than an enamel shell. Restoration

4 day diet analysis sheet for...... John Smith ....

	Thursday Time	Thursday Item	Friday Time	Friday Item	Saturday Time	Saturday Item	Sunday Time	Sunday Item
Before breakfast			7.00	2 cups of tea with 2 sugars	7.30	4 chocolate biscuits tea with 2 sugars		
Breakfast	8.30	sausages pitta bread ketchup tea with 2 sugars	8.30	banana			8.00	chocolate puffed rice breakfast cereal 1 glass cola drink
Morning	9.20 / 11.15	1 glass cola drink hot chocolate / chocolate bar	9.30	mug hot chocolate packet crisps can of diet cola drink	11.00	1 slice cherry cake	10.30	4 slices toast and peanut butter 1 piece cake
Mid-day meal	12.30	turkey salad sandwich 1 glass cola drink tea with 2 sugars	1.00 pm	2 pieces cheese on toast, garlic sausage 1 slice cake 1 glass cola drink	12.30	1 slice cake tea with 2 sugars	1.00 pm	fish pie 1 glass cola drink
Afternoon	4.00 pm	fizzy drink chocolate bar 1 slice cake	4.30 pm / 5.00 pm	ham 1 piece cake tea with 2 sugars / 1 glass cola drink	3.00 pm	sausages, beans, toast. an orange 1 can cola drink	2.00 pm / 4.30 pm / 6.00 pm	tea with 2 sugars 1 biscuit / 1 piece cake tea with 2 sugars / bar of chocolate
Evening meal	6.00 pm	salad, garlic sausage, ham, coleslaw	7.30 pm	burger and chips 1 can of cola drink	8.00 pm	spagehetti bolognaise ice cream	9.00 pm	fish and chips, peas 1 glass cola drink
Evening	10.30 pm	sausages crisps 1 glass fizzy drink			9.30 pm	tea with 2 sugars		

Fig. 1.4 The patient's diet sheet.

Table 1.3 Dietary advice

Aims	Methods
Reduce the amount of sugar	Check manufacturers' labels and avoid foods with sugars such as sucrose, glucose and fructose listed early in the ingredients. Natural sugars (e.g. honey, brown sugar) are as cariogenic as purified or added sugars. When sweet foods are required, choose those containing sweetening agents such as saccharin, acesulfame-K and aspartame. Diet formulations contain less sugar than their standard counterparts. Reduce the sweetness of drinks and foods. Become accustomed to a less sweet diet overall.
Restrict frequency of sugar intakes to meal times as far as possible	Try to reduce snacking. When snacks are required select 'safe snacks' such as cheese, crisps, fruit or sugar-free sweets, such as mints or chewing gum (which not only has no sugar but also stimulates salivary flow and increases plaque pH). Use artificial sweeteners in drinks taken between meals.
Speed clearance of sugars from the mouth	Never finish meals with a sugary food or drink. Follow sugary foods with a sugar-free drink, chewing gum or a protective food such as cheese.

of such teeth with amalgam would require removal of all the unsupported, undermined enamel leaving little more than a root stump and a few spurs of tooth tissue. Restoration could be better achieved with a radiopaque glass ionomer and composite hybrid restoration. The glass ionomer used to replace the missing dentine must be radiopaque so that it is not confused with residual or secondary caries on radiographs. A composite linked to dentine with a bonding agent would be an alternative to the glass ionomer.

■ *Figure 1.5 shows the restored lower first molar 2 months after endodontic treatment. What do you see and what long-term problem is evident?*

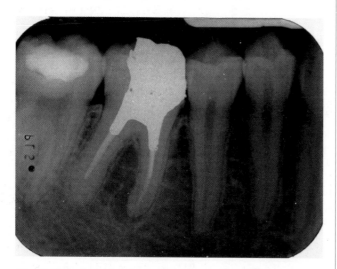

Fig. 1.5 Periapical radiograph of the restored lower first molar.

There is good bone healing around the apices and in the bifurcation. Complete healing would be expected after 6 months to 1 year at which time the success of root treatment can be judged.

As noted in the initial radiographs, the lower right first molar has lost its mesial contact, drifted and tilted. This makes it impossible to restore the normal contour of the mesial surface and contact point. The mesial surface is flat and there is no defined contact point. In the long term there is a risk of caries of the distal surface of the second premolar, and the caries is likely to affect a wider area of tooth and extend further gingivally than caries below a normal contact. The area will also be difficult to clean and there is a risk of localized periodontitis. Tilting of the occlusal surface may also favour food packing into the contact unless the contour of the restoration includes an artificially enhanced marginal ridge.

This tooth may require a crown in the long term. Much of the enamel is undermined and the tooth is weakened by endodontic treatment. A crown would allow the contact to have a better contour but the problem is insoluble while the tooth remains in its present position. Orthodontic uprighting could be considered.

■ *Why not simply extract the lower molar?*

Extraction of the lower right first molar may well be the preferred treatment. The caries is extensive, restoration of the tooth will be complex and expensive and problems will probably ensue in the long term. The missing tooth might not be readily visible.

To a large degree the decision will depend on the patient's wishes. If he would be happy with an edentulous space, the extraction appears an attractive proposition. However, if a restoration is required, a bridge will require preparation of two further teeth. A denture-based replacement is probably not indicated but an implant might be considered at a later date. Any hesitancy or uncertainty on the patient's part might well influence you to propose extraction.

Another factor affecting the decision is the condition and long-term prognosis of the other molars. If further molars are likely to be lost in the short or medium term it makes sense to conserve whichever teeth can be successfully restored.

CASE 2

A multilocular radiolucency

Summary

A 45-year-old African man presents in the Accident and Emergency department with an enlarged jaw. You must make a diagnosis and decide on treatment.

HISTORY

Complaint

The patient's main complaint is that his lower back teeth on the right side are loose and that his jaw on the right feels enlarged.

History of complaint

The patient has been aware of the teeth slowly becoming looser over the previous 6 months. They seem to be 'moving' and are now at a different height from his front teeth, making eating difficult. He is also concerned that his jaw is enlarged and there seems to be reduced space for his tongue. He has recently had the lower second molar on the right extracted. It was also loose but extraction does not seem to have cured the swelling. Although not in pain, he has finally decided to seek treatment.

Medical history

He is otherwise fit and healthy.

EXAMINATION

Extraoral examination

He is a fit-looking man with no obvious facial asymmetry but a slight fullness of the lower border of the mandible on the right. Palpation beneath the right angle reveals a smooth rounded bony hard enlargement on the lingual aspect. Deep cervical lymph nodes are palpable on the right side. They are only slightly enlarged, soft, not tender and freely mobile.

Intraoral examination

Intraoral examination reveals a large swelling of the right body of the mandible, mostly on the lingual side, extending from the first molar posteriorly to the angle. The second premolar and first molar are both mobile (grade III mobility) and over-erupted. Their occlusal surfaces are approximately 2–3 mm above the occlusal height of the remaining mandibular teeth. There is a medium-sized occlusal amalgam restoration in the first molar. All the posterior teeth in the maxilla on the right are missing, presumed extracted. The oral mucosa covering the enlarged part of the mandible appears normal. Oral hygiene is reasonable and gingival tissues appear healthy.

The teeth in the lower right quadrant all respond positively to testing for vitality.

■ *On the basis of what you know so far, what types of conditions would you consider to be present here?*

The history suggests a relatively slow-growing lesion, which is therefore likely to be benign. While this is not a definitive relationship, there are no specific features suggesting malignancy, such as perforation of the cortex, soft tissue mass, ulceration of the mucosa, numbness of the lip or devitalization of teeth. The character of the lymph node enlargement does not suggest malignancy.

The commonest jaw lesions which cause expansion are the odontogenic cysts. The commonest odontogenic cysts are the radicular (apical inflammatory) cyst, dentigerous cyst and odontogenic keratocyst. If this is a radicular cyst it could have arisen from the first molar, though the occlusal amalgam is relatively small and there seems no reason to suspect that the tooth is nonvital. A residual radicular cyst arising on the extracted second or third molars would be a possibility. A dentigerous cyst could be the cause if the third molar is unerupted. The possibility of an odontogenic keratocyst seems unlikely, because these cysts do not normally cause much expansion. An odontogenic tumour is a possible cause and an ameloblastoma would be the most likely one, because it is the commonest, and arises most frequently at this site and in this age group. There is a higher incidence in Africans. An ameloblastoma is much more likely than an odontogenic cyst to displace the teeth and make them grossly mobile. A giant cell granuloma and numerous other lesions are possibilities but are all less likely.

INVESTIGATIONS

■ *Radiographs are obviously indicated. Which views would you choose? Why?*

Several different views are necessary to show the full extent of the lesion. These could include:

View	Reason
Panoramic tomograph or an oblique lateral	To show the lesion from the lateral aspect. The oblique lateral would provide the better resolution but might not cover the anterior extent of this large lesion. The panoramic tomograph would provide a useful survey of the rest of the jaws but only that part of this expansile lesion in the line of the arch will be in focus. An oblique lateral view was taken.
A posterior–anterior (PA) of the jaws	To show the extent of mediolateral expansion of the posterior body, angle or ramus.
A lower true (90°) occlusal	To show the lingual expansion which will not be visible in the PA jaws view because of superimposition of the anterior body of the mandible.
A periapical of the lower right second premolar and first molar	To assess bone support and possible root resorption.

■ *These four different views are shown in Figures 2.1–2.4. Describe the radiographic features of the lesion.*

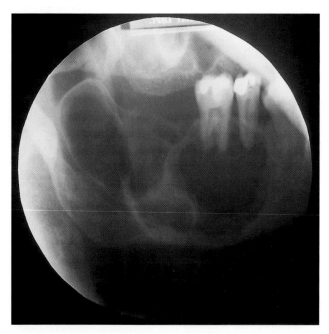

Fig. 2.1 Oblique lateral view.

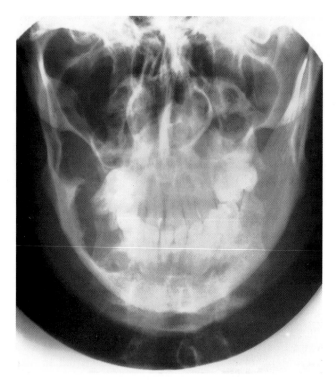

Fig. 2.2 Posterior–anterior view of the jaws.

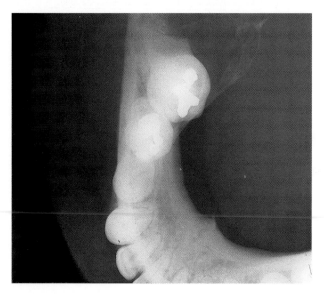

Fig. 2.3 Lower true occlusal view.

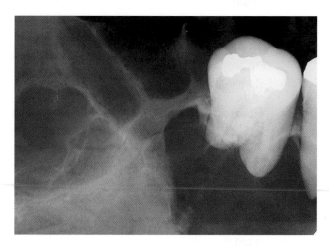

Fig. 2.4 Periapical view of the lower right first permanent molar.

Feature	Radiographic finding
Site	Posterior body, angle and ramus of the right mandible
Size	Large, about 10×8 cm, extending from the second premolar, back to the angle and involving all of the ramus up to the sigmoid notch, and from the expanded upper border of the alveolar bone down to the inferior dental canal.
Shape	Multilocular, producing the *soap bubble* appearance.
Outline/edge	Smooth, well defined and mostly well corticated.
Relative radiodensity	Radiolucent with distinct radiopaque septa producing the multilocular appearance. There is no evidence of separate areas of calcification within the lesion.
Effects on adjacent structures	Gross lingual expansion of mandible, but with minimal expansion of the buccal/lateral mandibular outline. Marked expansion of the superior margin of the alveolar bone and the anterior margin of the ascending ramus. The involved teeth have also been displaced superiorly. The roots of the involved teeth are slightly resorbed, but not as markedly as suggested by the periapical view. The lingual cortex does not appear to be perforated.

■ *Why do the roots of the first molar and second premolar appear to be so resorbed in the periapical view when the oblique lateral view shows minimal root resorption?*

The teeth are foreshortened because they lie at an angle to the film. This film has been taken using the bisected angle technique and several factors contribute to the distortion:
- the teeth have been displaced by the lesion, so the crowns lie more lingually, and the roots more buccally;
- the lingual expansion of the jaw makes film packet placement difficult, so it has had to be severely angulated away from the root apices;
- failure to take account of these two factors when positioning and angling the X-ray tubehead.

RADIOLOGICAL DIFFERENTIAL DIAGNOSIS

■ *What is your principal differential diagnosis?*

1. Ameloblastoma
2. Giant cell lesion

■ *Justify this differential diagnosis.*

Ameloblastoma classically produces an expansile multilocular radiolucency at the angle of the mandible.

As noted above, it most commonly presents at the age of this patient and is commoner in his racial group. The radiographs show the typical multilocular radiolucency, containing several large cystic spaces separated by bony septa, and the root resorption and tooth displacement and marked expansion are all consistent with an ameloblastoma of this size.

A giant cell lesion. A central giant cell granuloma is possible. Lesions can arise at almost any age but the radiological features and site are slightly different, making ameloblastoma the preferred diagnosis. Central giant cell granuloma produces an expansile and sometimes apparently multilocular radiolucency, but there would be no root resorption and the lesion may be less radiolucent (because it consists of solid tissue rather than cystic neoplasm), often containing wispy osteoid or fine bone septa subdividing the

lesion into a *honeycomb* like pattern. However, these typical features are not always seen. The spectrum of radiological appearances ranges from lesions which mimic odontogenic and solitary bone cysts to those which appear identical to ameloblastoma or other odontogenic tumours. The aneurysmal bone cyst is another giant cell lesion which could produce this radiographic appearance with prominent expansion. Adjacent teeth are usually displaced but rarely resorbed. However, aneurysmal bone cyst is much rarer in the jaws than central giant cell granuloma.

■ *What types of lesions are less likely and why?*

Several lesions remain possible but are less likely either on the basis of their features or relative rarity.

Rarer odontogenic tumours including particularly odontogenic fibroma and myxoma. These similar benign connective tissue odontogenic tumours are often indistinguishable from one another radiographically. Odontogenic myxoma is commoner than fibroma but both are relegated to the position of unlikely diagnoses on the basis of their relative rarity and the younger age group affected. Both usually cause unilocular or apparently multilocular expansile radiolucencies at the angle of the mandible which displace adjacent teeth or sometimes loosen or resorb them. A characteristic, though inconsistent feature is that the internal dividing septa are usually fine and arranged at right angles to one another, in a pattern sometimes said to resemble the letters 'X' and 'Y' or the strings of a tennis racket. In myxoma, septa can also show the bubbly *honeycomb* pattern described in giant cell granuloma.

Odontogenic keratocyst. This is unlikely to be the cause of this lesion but in view of its relative frequency it might still be included at the end of the differential diagnosis. It should be included because it can cause a large multilocular radiolucency at the angle of the mandible in adults, usually slightly younger than this patient. However, the growth pattern of an odontogenic keratocyst is quite different from the present lesion. Odontogenic keratocysts usually extend a considerable distance into the body and/or ramus before causing significant expansion. Even when expansion is evident, it is usually a broad-based enlargement rather than a localized expansile mass. Adjacent teeth are rarely resorbed or displaced.

■ *What lesions have you discounted and why?*

Dentigerous cyst is a common cause of large radiolucent lesions at the angle of the mandible. However, the present lesion is not unilocular and does not contain an unerupted tooth. Similarly, the **radicular cyst** is unilocular but associated with a non-vital tooth.

Malignant neoplasms, either primary or metastatic. As noted above, the clinical features do not suggest malignancy and the radiographs show an apparently benign, slowly enlarging lesion.

FURTHER INVESTIGATIONS

■ *Is a biopsy required?*

Yes. If the lesion is an ameloblastoma the treatment will be excision, whereas if it is a giant cell granuloma curettage will be sufficient. A definitive diagnosis based on biopsy is required.

■ *Would aspiration biopsy be helpful?*

No. If odontogenic keratocyst were suspected, this diagnosis might be confirmed by aspirating keratin. It would also be helpful in trying to decide whether the lesion were solid or cystic. It would not be particularly helpful in the diagnosis of ameloblastoma.

■ *What precautions would you take at biopsy?*

An attempt should be made to obtain a sample of solid lesion. If this is an ameloblastoma and an expanded area of jaw is selected for biopsy it will almost certainly overlie a cyst in the neoplasm. A large part of many ameloblastomas is cyst space and the stretched cyst lining is not always sufficiently characteristic histologically to make the diagnosis. If the lesion proves to be cystic on biopsy, the surgeon should open up the cavity and explore it to identify solid tumour for sampling.
    The surgical access must be carefully closed on bone to ensure that healing is uneventful and infection does not develop in the cyst spaces. The expanded areas may be covered by only a thin layer of *eggshell* periosteal bone. Once this is opened it may be difficult to replace the margin of a flap on bone.

■ *The histological appearances of the biopsy are shown in Figures 2.5 and 2.6. What do you see?*

The specimen is stained with haematoxylin and eosin. At low power the lesion is seen to consist of islands of epithelium separated by thin pink collagenous bands. Each island has a prominent outer layer of basal cells, a paler staining zone within that, and sometimes a pink keratinized zone of cells centrally. One of the islands shows early cyst formation. At

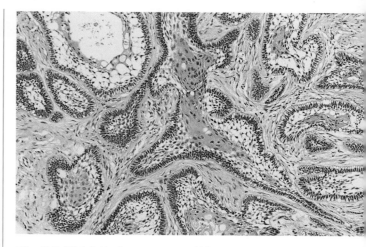

Fig. 2.5 Histological appearance of biopsy at low power.

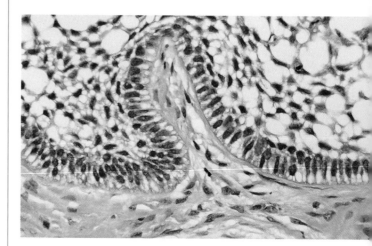

Fig. 2.6 Histological appearance of biopsy at high power.

higher power, the outer basal cell layer is seen to comprise elongated palisaded cells with reversed nuclear polarity (nuclei placed away from the basement membrane). Towards the basement membrane many of the cells have a clear cytoplasmic zone and the overall appearance looks like piano keys. Above the basal cell layer is a zone of very loosely packed stellate cells with large spaces between them. There is no inflammation.

■ *How do you interpret these appearances?*

The appearances are typical and diagnostic of ameloblastoma. The elongated basal cells bear a superficial resemblance to preameloblasts and the looser cells to stellate reticulum. The arrangement of the epithelium in islands with the stellate reticulum in their centres constitutes the follicular pattern of ameloblastoma.

DIAGNOSIS

The final diagnosis is ameloblastoma, of the follicular pattern.

TREATMENT

■ *What treatment will be required?*

The ameloblastoma is classified as a benign neoplasm. However, it is locally invasive and in some cases permeates the medullary cavity around the main tumour margin. Ameloblastoma should be excised with a 1-cm margin of normal bone and around any suspected perforations in the cortex. If ameloblastoma has escaped from the medullary cavity, it may spread extensively in the soft tissues and requires excision with an even larger margin. The lower border of the mandible may be intact and is sometimes left in place to avoid the need for full thickness resection of the mandible and a bone graft. This causes a low risk of recurrence, but such recurrences are slow-growing and may be dealt with conservatively after the main portion of the mandible has healed. The fact that the ameloblastoma is of the follicular pattern is of no significance for treatment.

■ *What other imaging investigations would be appropriate for this patient?*

In order to plan the resection accurately, the extent of the tumour and any cortical perforations must be identified. Computed tomography (CT) and/or magnetic resonance imaging (MRI) would show the full extent of the lesion in bone and surrounding soft tissue respectively.

CASE 3

Gingival recession

Summary

A 30-year-old woman has gingival recession. Assess her condition and discuss treatment options.

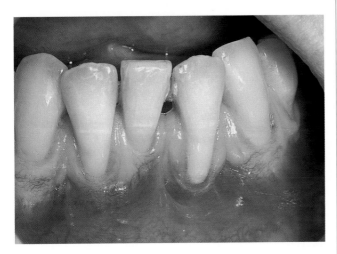

Fig. 3.1 The appearance of the lower incisors.

HISTORY

Complaint

The patient is worried about the gingival recession around her lower front teeth which she feels is worsening.

History of complaint

She remembers noticing the recession for at least the previous 5 years. She thinks it has worsened over the last 12 months. There has recently been some sensitivity to hot and cold and gingival soreness, most noticeably on toothbrushing or eating ice cream.

Dental history

The patient has been a patient of your practice for about 10 years and you have discussed her recession at previous visits and reassured her. She has a low caries rate and generally good oral hygiene.

Medical history

She is a fit and healthy individual and is not a smoker.

■ *What further specific questions would you ask to help identify a possible cause?*

How often do you brush your teeth? Provided brushing is effective, cleaning once a day is sufficient to maintain gingival health. However, most patients clean two or three times each day and some brush excessively in terms of frequency, duration and force used. Trauma from brushing is considered a factor in some patients' recession, and recession may indicate a need to reduce the frequency and duration of cleaning while maintaining its effectiveness. In this instance the patient has a normal toothbrushing habit but should clean no more than twice each day and for a sensible period of time.

Have you had orthodontic treatment? A lower incisor is missing, suggesting that some intervention may have taken place. Fixed orthodontics in the lower labial segment is occasionally associated with gingival recession in patients with thin buccal gingiva, narrow alveolar processes and correction of severe crowding. Plaque control may be compromised during the wearing of an orthodontic appliance and, even over a relatively short period, this can contribute to the problem. In this instance the patient had undergone extraction of the incisor but had not worn an appliance.

EXAMINATION

Intraoral examination

■ *The appearance of the lower incisors is shown in Figure 3.1. What do you see?*

— Missing lower left central incisor.
— Unrestored teeth.
— No plaque is visible except for a small amount at the cervical margin of the lower left lateral incisor.
— Gingival recession affecting all lower incisors and, to a lesser extent, the lower canines
— Apart from the abnormal contour, the buccal gingivae are pink and healthy and the interdental papillae are normal.
— Reduction in width of keratinized (cornified) attached gingival epithelium. In places, attached gingiva appears absent.

■ *What clinical assessments would you make, how would you make them and why are they important?*

See Table 3.1.

On performing these clinical examinations you find that all probing depths are 1–2 mm with no bleeding. The width of keratinized gingiva varies with the degree of recession. The lower left lateral incisor has no attached gingiva and tension on the lip displaces the gingival margin. No teeth have increased mobility and no possible occlusal factors are present. There is no reason to suspect loss of vitality and all teeth respond to testing.

Table 3.1 Clinical assessments in patient with gingival recession

Assessment	Method	Importance
Recession	Measure from the gingival margin to the cement-enamel junction	Provides baseline readings to assess progression
Probing depths	Routine periodontal probing	Detects associated loss of attachment undermining the reduced width of attached gingiva
Bleeding on probing	Routine recording of bleeding on probing; immediate or delayed	Indicates the presence of gingival inflammation and poor oral hygiene
Amount of attached gingiva	Subtract the probing depth recording from the width of keratinized gingiva	Gives the amount of apparent attached gingiva bound down to bone and thus functional
Presence of functional attached gingiva	Pull gently on the lip or depress the labial sulcus mucosa, placing tension on the attached gingiva or gingival margin	If the gingival margin is displaced from the teeth or is otherwise mobile there is inadequate functional width of attached gingiva, regardless of its absolute measurement
Tooth mobility	Try to displace teeth in a buccolingual direction using two instrument handles. Fingers are too compressible to do this effectively	Important if teeth are very mobile, but not a very useful diagnostic or prognostic indicator with small amounts of buccal recession only
Vitality testing	Routine methods: electronic pulp tester or hot/cold	Nonvital teeth are compromised and this needs to be taken into account in treatment planning.
Occlusion	Direct examination of intercuspal position and excursive contacts	If a traumatic overbite is present it may cause or exacerbate recession

INVESTIGATIONS

■ *What radiographs are indicated?*

Radiographs would give little additional information. The degree of bone loss on the buccal aspect, including bone dehiscence and fenestrations, is not well shown on radiographs because of superimposition of the roots. Radiographs might help if interdental bone loss is suspected, but the intact interdental papillae, together with minimal probing depths, suggest normal interdental bone height. A radiograph would be of value if mobility indicated a need to assess root length and bone height.

DIAGNOSIS

■ *What is your diagnosis and what is the likely aetiology?*

The patient has gingival recession. In this case the assessment has not provided a diagnosis any more accurate than that given by the patient but the features should give some clues to the possible aetiology.

Recession is probably multifactorial in aetiology. The most important factor is probably anatomical variation between patients. Some individuals have very thin gingival tissue buccally, both soft tissue and bone. When the buccal plate of the alveolus is thin, bony dehiscence or fenestrations below the soft tissue are more likely. For these reasons, there is more recession on the teeth which are prominent in the arch and least on slightly instanding teeth (see the more instanding central incisor in Figure 3.1). When these predisposing factors are present, other insults become important. The most important is probably traumatic toothbrushing. Plaque-induced marginal inflammation will also destroy the thin tissue at this site relatively quickly. Traumatic occlusion may also contribute.

In this case the patient is maintaining a very good standard of plaque control and there is no cervical abrasion which might be further evidence of toothbrush trauma.

■ *What advice and treatment would you provide?*

- Ensure a sensible, atraumatic but effective brushing regime to remove the small amount of plaque present and explain the importance of good oral hygiene in areas of recession.
- Reassure the patient that the condition is not necessarily progressive, though it is irreversible.
- Monitor for progression with the aid of clinical measurements. A drawing, clinical photographs or study casts are very helpful and should be repeated at intervals.
- Treat the dentine hypersensitivity. Recession alone should not be painful. Ensure that the exposed root surface is suffering neither early caries nor erosion. Check the diet for sugars, acid drinks and foods and apply topical antihypersensitivity agents. This is another reason to perfect the oral hygiene around these teeth.

In this case the patient maintained good plaque control but the recession worsened slowly over a period of several years until there was a lack of functional attached gingiva.

■ *What other treatments might be possible? Are they effective?*

Table 3.2 shows alternative treatments.

In this case a free gingival graft was placed and the result is shown in Figure 3.2.

Table 3.2 Alternative treatment

Treatment	Effectiveness
Mucogingival surgery to correct the recession, either a lateral pedicle graft, double papilla flap, or a coronally repositioned flap. These may be used in conjunction with an interpositional (subepithelial connective tissue) graft. These are essentially cosmetic operations.	May be effective in carefully selected cases. The presence of adjacent interdental papillae and suitable donor sites is essential. Total root coverage is difficult to achieve and unpredictable, especially in the long term.
Mucogingival surgery to provide a wider and functional zone of attached gingiva. This therapeutic procedure provides a zone of thicker tissue which is more resistant to further recession and less prone to soreness with normal brushing. A free gingival graft is the treatment of choice.	Highly effective. Grafting palatal mucosa into the alveolar mucosa prevents the lip pulling the gingiva from the teeth. Even if the gingival margin has little attached gingiva, it can remain healthy if protected from displacement or other trauma.
Provision of a thin acrylic gingival stent or veneer.	Can provide excellent cosmetic result if well made, but only considered for extensive recession in highly visible areas. The usual indication is the upper incisors following periodontal surgery with loss of papillae. Rarely used and not applicable to this case.

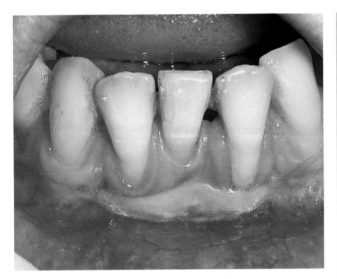

Fig. 3.2 Appearance of the free gingival graft 6 months after placement.

■ *What do you see; is the graft successful?*

Yes, the graft appears successful. Palatal connective tissue and overlying epithelium has been placed apical to the lower incisor gingival margin to provide a wider zone of attached keratinized gingiva. Because the palatal connective tissue is transferred the epithelium retains its keratinized palate structure.

■ *Does the graft need to lie at the gingival margin?*

No. The graft forms the gingival margin on the lower left lateral incisor but elsewhere lies below the margin. Provided the graft is firmly bound down to the underlying tissue it will stabilize the gingival margin against displacement on lip movement.

■ *Why not place the graft over the root as well and correct the recession?*

As noted in the table above, surgery to correct the recession itself is difficult to achieve and unpredictable, especially in the

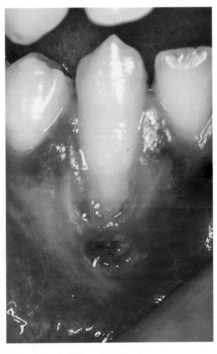

Fig. 3.3 A different patient.

long term. The root surface does not provide a nutrient bed on which the free graft can survive. Grafts in this situation would have to be pedicled to ensure their nutrient supply and also need to be placed so that they receive some nutrient from an adjacent exposed connective tissue bed. A more predictable result may be obtained by using an interpositional (subepithelial) connective tissue graft. A free graft is most unlikely to be successful if simply placed over the root surface.

■ *Figure 3.3 shows a different patient with recession. What does the appearance tell you?*

There is approximately 4 mm of recession buccally on the lower right canine. Apical to the gingival margin there is a hole in the gingival tissue. Plaque and subgingival calculus (formed within a periodontal pocket) are visible and the tissue is inflamed. The small 'bridge' of tissue at the gingival margin is not attached to the tooth surface and will eventually break down. In this case the recession is secondary to pocket formation in a plaque-induced periodontitis. Inflammation associated with subgingival calculus has caused loss of much of the buccal bone.

■ *How would treatment of this patient's recession differ?*

It would differ only in the early stages. Inflammation must be treated by oral hygiene improvement and subgingival debridement. If, after a period to allow healing, there is resolution of inflammation, the situation is very similar to that in the first case and assessment and treatment would be identical. There would be no value in attempting to surgically correct the fenestration in the attached gingiva. As discussed above, grafting onto the root surface is technically complex and success is unpredictable.

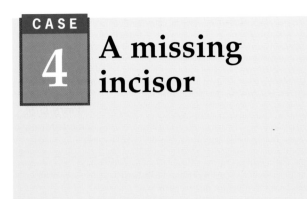

CASE 4
A missing incisor

Summary

A 9-year-old boy is referred to you in the orthodontic department with an unerupted upper left central incisor. What is the cause and how may it be treated?

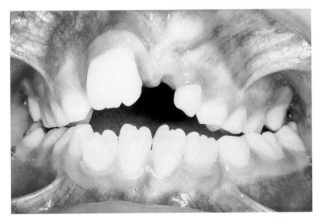

Fig. 4.1 The appearance of the patient on presentation.

HISTORY

Complaint

The patient's upper left central incisor has not erupted although he is 9 years old. His mother is very concerned about her son's appearance and is anxious for him to be treated.

History of complaint

The upper left deciduous predecessor had been present until about 4 months ago. It was extracted by the patient's general dental practitioner in an attempt to speed up the eruption of the permanent successor. Despite this, there has been no change in appearance. The upper permanent central incisor on the opposite side erupted normally at 7 years of age.

Medical history

The patient has suffered from asthma since he was 4 years old. This is controlled using Ventolin.

EXAMINATION

Extraoral examination

There are no extraoral signs or symptoms and the patient is an active, happy boy.

Intraoral examination

- *The appearance of the mouth is shown in Figure 4.1. What do you see?*

The patient is in the early mixed dentition stage and the teeth present are:

$$\frac{6EDCB1 \mid BCDE6}{6EDC21 \mid 12\ DE6}$$

No upper left central incisor is present, but there is a pale swelling high in the upper labial sulcus above the edentulous space and the upper left B. There has been some loss of space in the region of the absent upper central incisor.

There is a tendency to an anterior open bite which is slightly more pronounced on the right.

There is mild upper and lower arch crowding and a unilateral crossbite on the left. If you were able to examine the patient you would discover that this is associated with a lateral displacement of the mandibular position. The lower centre line is shifted to the left.

There are no restorations but the mouth is not very clean.

- *What are the possible causes of an apparently absent upper central incisor?*

The incisor may be missing or have failed to erupt. Possible causes include the following:

Missing	Developmentally absent
	Extracted
	Avulsed
Failure to erupt	Dilaceration and/or displacement as a result of trauma
	Scar tissue preventing eruption
	Supernumerary tooth preventing eruption
	Insufficient space as a result of crowding
	Pathological lesion (e.g. cyst or odontogenic tumour)

- *What specific questions would you ask the parents?*

The most important questions are related to trauma. Avulsion or dilaceration would follow significant trauma which is likely to be recalled by the parent. The parent should be asked whether the deciduous predecessor was discoloured. If it was this would provide evidence of loss of vitality, perhaps related to trauma. Extraction would be unusual and a cause should be readily obtained in the history.

In response to your questioning the parent reports that the patient fell on his face when he was much younger. At the time of the accident there was considerable injury to his lips and teeth, but no tooth loss was noticed and no dental opinion was sought.

- *What are the likely causes of the anterior open bite and shift in the lower centre line?*

The anterior open bite is probably associated with a thumb-sucking or similar habit. The shift in the centre line is probably caused by the combination of crowding and early exfoliation of the lower left C.

■ *Give a differential diagnosis for the cause of the missing incisor. Explain each possibility.*

Dilaceration of the central incisor as a result of the injury appears the most likely cause. However, it is unclear whether the injury was severe enough to cause dilaceration. Dilaceration usually follows intrusion and the intruded tooth might well have re-erupted into its normal position. The swelling in the sulcus does not lie on the normal eruption path of the central incisor, and dilaceration could explain the abnormal position.

A supernumerary tooth or an odontome would be the next most likely possibility if trauma is not the cause. Supernumerary teeth are not uncommon in the premaxilla (1–3% of the population), and the late-forming (tuberculate) type which often lies adjacent to the crown of the permanent incisor frequently causes delay or failure of eruption.

A pathological lesion appears unlikely but cannot be excluded. There is no evidence of alveolar expansion to suggest a cyst, which would be the most likely cause and could arise from the tooth itself, a supernumerary or an odontome. An unexpected lesion remains a remote possibility.

■ *What causes have you excluded and why?*

Crowding appears to be an unlikely cause. It would have to be very severe to cause a delay of up to 2 years and this patient's teeth are only mildly crowded. Crowding is a very unusual cause for failure of eruption of a central incisor because loss of the B would provide enough space for eruption.

Scarring of the alveolus delays eruption because it slows resorption of bone over the tooth and because fibrosis and thickening of the mucoperiosteum resists tooth movement. This is an unlikely cause because there is no reason to suspect scarring, the deciduous predecessor having been extracted only 4 months ago.

Avulsion can be excluded because it seems that the tooth has never erupted and there is no recent history of trauma.

Developmental causes of absence appear most unlikely. The swelling in the upper sulcus would seem to indicate that the tooth is present but has failed to erupt. A missing central incisor without other missing teeth would be an extremely rare finding.

INVESTIGATIONS

Radiographs are required to determine whether or not the unerupted tooth is present, to establish whether it is the cause of the swelling in the sulcus and detect possible supernumerary teeth.

■ *What radiographic views would you request and why?*

See Table 4.1.

The radiographs of the patient are shown in Figures 4.2–4.4.

■ *What do the radiographs show?*

The panoramic tomograph confirms the presence of a full complement of developing permanent successors, excluding the third molars which would not be expected to have formed. However, a crypt should be present between the ages of $8\frac{1}{2}$ and 10 years of age and there is a suggestion of early crypt formation in the lower left quadrant. The unerupted permanent upper left central incisor is clearly visible on this radiograph and its shape is not normal but the root shape cannot be seen. It is not possible to establish the labiopalatal position of the tooth in this film nor to detect an adjacent supernumerary tooth which may lie outside the tomographic focal trough.

The periapical view gives considerably more detail. The upper left central incisor has an intact but distorted root. Its apical development appears normal and similar to that of the right central incisor but the foreshortened appearance suggests dilaceration. Using this film in conjunction with the panoramic view and applying the principle of vertical parallax you can see that the crown of the central incisor is labially positioned. This is consistent with the swelling in the sulcus being caused by the crown of the tooth. No supernumerary tooth is present.

The lateral view completes the picture and shows clearly the displaced crown of the central incisor. From the three films it is possible to deduce that the crown and root of the tooth are misaligned, the crown deflected labially with its incisal edge pointing forwards into the labial sulcus and the root developing in the normal direction.

■ *What is your final diagnosis?*

The upper left central incisor is dilacerated, probably as a result of intrusion of the deciduous predecessor in the injury sustained in infancy.

TREATMENT

■ *What are the options for treatment?*

If the dilaceration were severe the tooth would require extraction. Then either of the following options could be selected:
1. Align the adjacent teeth, ideally with fixed appliances, using the central incisor space. The lateral incisor would replace the central incisor and could be masked to simulate it. In the short term this could be accomplished by adhesive restoration but in the longer term a permanent restoration would be necessary. The canine might also need restoration or masking so that it would not appear incongruous, especially in a patient with slender lateral incisors. This option is not ideal because the final appearance is often poor.
2. Immediate replacement of the extracted central incisor by a denture or adhesive bridge with permanent restoration or possibly a single tooth implant in adulthood (see Case 23).

If, on the radiographs, the dilaceration does not appear to be too severe or lies in the apical portion of the root, consideration could be given to aligning the tooth

Table 4.1 Radiographic views and their purposes

View	Reason
Dental panoramic tomograph	To provide a general view of the developing dentition and establish the presence or absence of the permanent teeth
Upper standard occlusal or periapicals of the edentulous area, taken with a paralleling technique	To provide a more detailed view of the region, in particular the root morphology and any adjacent structures such as supernumerary teeth or pathological lesions. These may lie outside the focal trough of the tomograph or be obscured by superimposition of other structures in the panoramic view. If periapical views are taken they should include the adjacent teeth in case these were damaged in the original accident. In addition the standard occlusal and panoramic view can be used together to establish the relationship of unerupted structures relative to the dental arch, using the principle of (vertical) parallax. Objects lying nearer to the X-ray tube (labially positioned) appear to move in the opposite direction to the tube relative to a fixed point. Those further away (palatally positioned) appear to move in the same direction as the tube.
A lateral view	Confirms the presence of any distortion of the tooth, if dilacerated, and confirms the relationship of the tooth to the labial swelling in a third dimension.

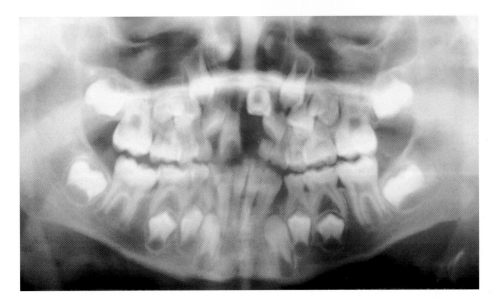

Fig. 4.2 Dental panoramic tomograph.

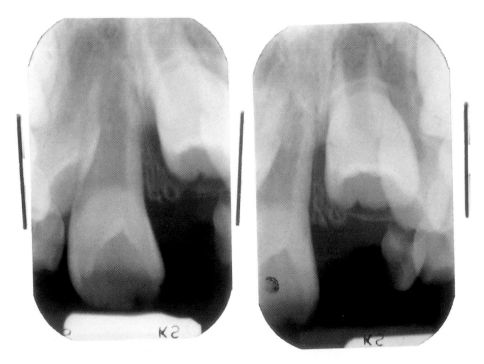

Fig. 4.3 Periapical views.

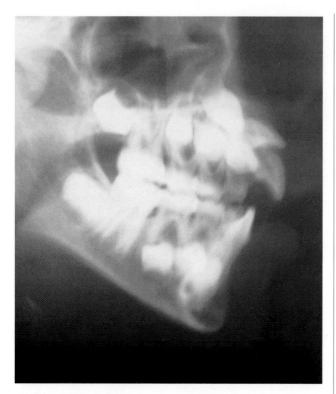

Fig. 4.4 Lateral view.

orthodontically. This would involve regaining any lost space followed by localized surgical exposure of the crown of the tooth and applying extrusive traction with an orthodontic appliance.

■ *What factors affect the selection of a particular treatment?*

- Position and severity of the dilaceration (see above)
- The size of overjet
- Degree of crowding
- Position and condition of the other permanent teeth
- The general condition of the mouth
- The attitude of the child and parent

■ *Assuming none of these factors prevents the ideal treatment, what would you recommend for this case?*

In this case the ideal treatment is to extrude and align the dilacerated tooth into the arch.

The dilaceration appears to be in the root and relatively mild. Therefore, an attempt should be made to regain the lost space to accommodate the central incisor crown. This would be best achieved by extraction of both upper Cs and the upper left B to encourage eruption of permanent lateral incisors. Some months later the dilacerated tooth should be surgically exposed and an orthodontic attachment with a length of gold chain placed on its palatal surface for extrusion.

■ *Should a fixed or removable appliance be used?*

As the tooth movements are relatively simple an upper removable appliance can be used at this stage. More control and more accurate tooth positioning would be achieved with a fixed appliance. However, the patient will probably require further fixed appliance treatment at a later age and the fine adjustment of tooth position could be performed then.

■ *Design a suitable removable appliance.*

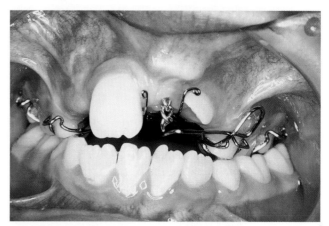

Fig. 4.5 The fitted extrusion appliance.

The appliance consists of:
— cribs on D|D (0.6-mm wire)
— cribs on 6|6 (0.7-mm wire)
— finger springs on 1| and |2 (0.5-mm wire) to retract and regain the space for the |1.
— a buccal arm to extrude |1 (0.7-mm wire) attached to the gold chain bonded to |1.

■ *Figure 4.6 shows the position of the dilacerated tooth after approximately 18 months of active treatment. What further treatment may be necessary at a later stage of dental development?*

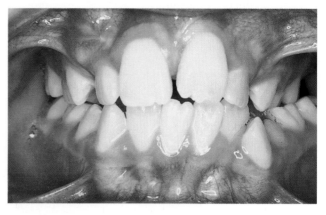

Fig. 4.6 After 18 months of treatment.

Ideally it would be appropriate to relieve the crowding in the permanent dentition and align the teeth, correcting the unilateral posterior crossbite and eliminating the mandibular displacement. Details of appropriate treatment cannot be finalized until the patient passes from mixed dentition to permanent dentition at about 10–12 years of age.

A dry mouth

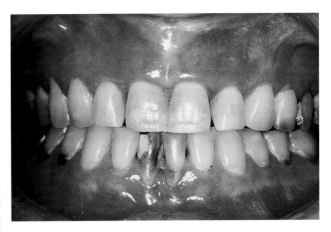
Fig. 5.1 Appearance of the patient's anterior teeth.

Summary

A 50-year-old lady presents to you in your hospital dental department complaining of dry mouth. Identify the cause and plan treatment.

HISTORY

Complaint

She complains of dryness which makes many aspects of her life a misery. The dryness is both uncomfortable and renders eating and speech difficult. She is forced to keep a bottle of water by her side at all times.

History of complaint

She first noticed the dry mouth about 4 or 5 years ago though it may have been present for longer. At first it was only an intermittent problem but over the last 3 years or so the dryness has become constant. Recently the mouth has become sore as well as dry.

Medical history

The patient describes herself as generally fit and well but has had to attend her medical practitioner for poor circulation in her fingers. They blanch rapidly in the cold and are painful on rewarming. She has also used artificial tears for dry eyes for the last 2 years but takes no other medication.

EXAMINATION

Extraoral examination

She is a well-looking lady without detectable cervical lymphadenopathy. There is no facial asymmetry or enlargement of the parotid glands and the sub-mandibular glands appear normal on bimanual palpation. Her eyes and fingers appear normal.

Intraoral examination

■ *The appearance of the patient's mouth is shown in Figures 5.1 and 5.2. What do you see? How do you interpret the findings?*

The alveolar mucosa appears 'glazed' and translucent or thin (atrophic) suggesting long-standing xerostomia. Some oral

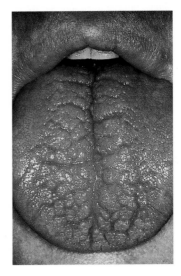
Fig. 5.2 Appearance of the patient's tongue.

debris adheres between the teeth, again suggesting dryness which causes plaque to be thicker and more tenacious. There are carious lesions and restorations at the cervical margins of the lower anterior teeth, indicating a high caries rate. The tongue is lobulated and fissured. Both features suggest a lack of saliva.

If you were able to examine the patient you would find her mouth does feel dry. Gloved fingers and mirror adhere to the mucosa making examination uncomfortable. Parts of the mucosa, especially the palate and dorsal tongue appear redder than normal. No saliva is pooling in the floor of the mouth and what saliva can be identified is frothy and thick. Small amounts of clear but viscid saliva can be expressed from all four main salivary ducts.

■ *What are the common and important causes of xerostomia and how are they subdivided?*

In true xerostomia the salivary flow is reduced. The term 'false xerostomia' describes the sensation of dryness despite normal salivary output.

Type of xerostomia	Common causes
False	Mouth breathing
	Mucosal disease
	Psychological
True	Drugs
	Dehydration
	Sjögren's syndrome
	Irradiation
	Neurological
	Developmental anomaly

■ *On the basis of the history and examination which cause is the most likely? Why?*

Sjögren's syndrome is the most likely cause. It is the commonest single medical disorder causing xerostomia. It also causes dry eyes and predominantly affects female patients of middle age. Sjögren's syndrome is sometimes defined by the presence of dry eyes and mouth, with or without an autoimmune/connective tissue disorder. This patient meets these criteria though they are rather imprecise and further investigations would be required to confirm the diagnosis.

■ *Which causes have you excluded and why?*

Drugs are by far the commonest cause of true xerostomia but this patient is not taking any medication.

Dehydration is a common cause in elderly people who may have a habitual low fluid intake, especially when institutionalized. It also accompanies cardiac or renal failure or diuretic drugs. (The combination of drugs and disease probably explains the apparent association of xerostomia with age.) These are not factors in this case.

False xerostomia is very common. Those who sleep with an open mouth will have xerostomia on waking, compounded by the normal reduction in salivary secretion at night. Diseases causing oral mucosal roughness such as lichen planus or candidiasis may cause a sensation of dryness but no such condition is present. False xerostomia may be a feature, sometimes a central one, in neurosis and psychosis. However, this patient's mouth is genuinely dry. The history of prolonged and unremitting dryness over a period of years almost always indicates salivary disorder and the appearance of the mucosa and the high caries rate indicate true xerostomia.

Neurological and developmental causes, such as aplasia of gland or atresia of ducts, are very rare and need not be considered further until common causes have been investigated. There is no history of irradiation of the head and neck.

■ *What is Sjögren's syndrome and how may the condition be subclassified?*

Sjögren's syndrome is a poorly understood autoimmune disorder in which exocrine glands are destroyed. In primary Sjögren's syndrome the salivary and lacrimal glands are those most affected (though there are often nonspecific systemic signs of autoimmune disease such as Raynaud's phenomenon) and there is sometimes salivary gland swelling. Other exocrine glands and organs are also affected. In secondary Sjögren's syndrome there is an accompanying connective tissue disorder such as rheumatoid arthritis, systemic lupus erythematosus or mixed connective tissue disease. Other exocrine glands are less severely affected in the secondary form, the mouth is usually less dry and salivary glands are very rarely enlarged.

INVESTIGATIONS

■ *What simple test differentiates false and true xerostomia?*

Measuring the whole saliva flow rate. This may be done by asking the patient to tilt their head forward to allow all saliva to flow into a graduated specimen container for 10 minutes. Although this patient is strongly suspected to have true xerostomia it would still be a useful test because it provides a baseline reading against which disease severity and progression may be judged.

When you measure the flow, the patient has a whole salivary flow rate of 0.1 ml/minute.

■ *What salivary flow rate would you consider to indicate xerostomia?*

Approximately 500 ml of saliva are secreted daily, mostly during eating and drinking, and very little at night. Rates vary greatly between individuals but less than 2 ml in 10 minutes (0.2 ml/minute) unstimulated whole saliva flow is generally considered to indicate xerostomia.

This patient has true xerostomia.

■ *What further investigations are required and why is each performed?*

Although a number of investigations will be required to confirm the diagnosis, the immediate problem is one of soreness. A dry mouth is not usually sore unless there is superimposed candidal infection. Smears, a saliva sample or a therapeutic trial of antifungal agent are required to exclude this possibility.

The diagnosis of Sjögren's syndrome is straightforward when the clinical presentation is florid, and may then be based on history and examination alone. However, numerous investigations are required in most patients with suspected Sjögren's syndrome in whom there are just a few early signs (Table 5.1). Many investigations are possible but only the minimum required to make the diagnosis need to be performed. A selection is usually necessary because every test will be negative in a small proportion of patients and none is completely specific.

Table 5.1 Investigations for patients with Sjögren's syndrome

Sample	Test	Relevance
Saliva	Whole salivary flow rate Culture for candidal count Stimulated parotid flow	See above; differentiates false from true xerostomia To exclude superimposed candidiasis Accurate estimation of maximum possible parotid salivary flow
Blood tests	Full blood picture Erythrocyte sedimentation rate (ESR) Immunoglobulin levels Autoantibody screen	Mild anaemia is common in all autoimmune conditions and may require treatment Relatively nonspecific but raised in inflammatory conditions, useful for monitoring their activity after treatment. Often raised in autoimmune disorders and may be markedly raised in primary Sjögren's syndrome Autoantibodies are a frequent finding in autoimmune disease. This appears to be a partly nonspecific effect and many different autoantibodies may be seen. The exact combination in the routine screen varies between centres but usually includes rheumatoid factor, antinuclear, antithyroid, antiparietal cell and antimitochondrial antibody. Additional autoantibodies which may be seen in Sjögren's syndrome are antisalivary gland duct antibody and ssA and ssB autoantibodies (anti-Ro and anti-La) directed against extractable nuclear antigens. None of these antibodies is individually helpful in diagnosis but the presence of more than one is typical. They may help diagnosis of connective tissue disease in secondary Sjögren's syndrome and ssA and ssB may indicate patients at risk of specific complications. Antisalivary gland duct antibody is not related to either the periductal infiltrates seen on biopsy or the pathogenesis of the disease.
Urine	Glucose	Occasionally useful to exclude unsuspected diabetes as a cause of dehydration.
Salivary gland	Sialogram Other imaging techniques Minor salivary gland biopsy Parotid gland biopsy	In established disease a sialogram almost always shows characteristic changes. Pertechnicate scintigraphy is a complex but useful test of secretion from individual glands. It is useful if sialography is not possible but involves a significant radiation dose. Magnetic resonance imaging is useful to delineate the extent of salivary gland swelling if present. The histological appearances of salivary glands are characteristic in established disease. Biopsy of major glands is difficult but the same changes may be seen in the minor glands of the lips and cheeks provided a sufficient sample is removed (6–8 glands). Biopsy of the tail of the parotid is possible without significant risk to branches of the facial nerve. It provides an excellent sample and may be useful when other techniques have failed or when other conditions need to be excluded. It may also be helpful in the diagnosis of lymphoma in swollen parotid glands. However, it is rarely performed.
Eye	Schirmer test Ophthalmological examination	This measures lacrimal secretion. Narrow filter paper strips are placed with one end under the lower eyelid and the length wetted after several minutes is recorded. In practice the test is not very reproducible. It is also uncomfortable and may cause corneal abrasions when the eye is very dry and for this reason is no longer recommended. Ophthalmological examination is preferable. Examination by an ophthalmologist using a slit lamp will detect conjunctival splits and Rose Bengal staining identifies dried tear secretion on the front of the eye. Though these changes are rarely helpful in diagnosis, examination and follow up is required to prevent long-term complications of dry eyes.

The results of this patient's investigations are:

Salivary culture	10 000 cfu *Candida sp.*/ml
Smear for candida	Hyphae present
Red cell indices	Normal
White cell count/differential count	Normal
Platelets	Normal
ESR	20 mm/hour
Ig levels	Normal
Autoantibodies	
Rose Waaler	Negative
RA latex	Negative
Antinuclear	Weak positive
Antithyroid	Negative
ssA	Positive
ssB	Positive
Urine glucose	Normal

■ **The parotid sialogram is shown in Figure 5.3. What do you see? What is your interpretation?**

The sialogram shows punctate sialectasis. The major duct is seen but almost no major or minor duct branches are visible. Small round spots of contrast medium are scattered throughout the gland, apparently unconnected with the duct tree. These features have some similarities to those in chronic nonspecific sialadenitis but are much more even and affect the whole gland equally. These features are characteristic of Sjögren's syndrome.

■ **The minor salivary gland biopsy is shown in Figures 5.4 and 5.5. What do you see?**

The low power view shows several minor salivary glands. A minimum of 6–8 glands is required for reliable diagnosis and

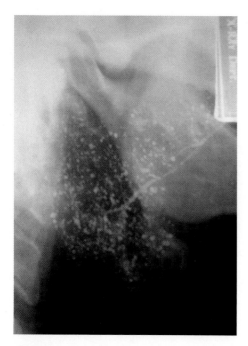

Fig. 5.3 Parotid sialogram.

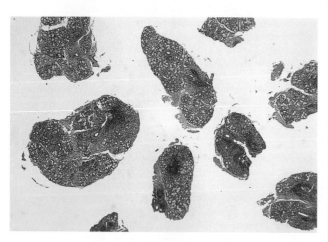

Fig. 5.4 Minor salivary gland biopsy; low power.

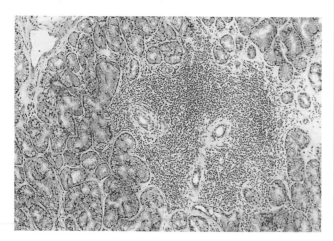

Fig. 5.5 Minor salivary gland biopsy; high power.

this sample is sufficient. Even at this low magnification, dark foci of inflammatory cells are visible (though they cannot be identified as such) and it can be seen that the lobular structure of the glands is largely intact.

The high power view shows one gland lobule. Centrally there are three small ducts surrounded by a dense lymphocytic infiltrate. The infiltrate is sharply defined and within the lymphocytic focus there is complete loss of acinar cells (acinar atrophy). Around the lymphocytes there is a zone of essentially normal uninflamed mucous salivary gland.

■ *How do you interpret these histological appearances?*

The focal lymphocytic sialadenitis centred on ducts and concentric sharply defined zones of acinar atrophy surrounded by normal acini are characteristic of Sjögren's syndrome.

DIAGNOSIS

■ *What is your final diagnosis?*

The patient has primary Sjögren's syndrome. The diagnosis was suspected on the basis of history and examination, and is confirmed by the characteristic sialogram and biopsy findings. The primary form of Sjögren's syndrome is indicated by the lack of autoimmune/connective tissue disease and the positivity for ssA and ssB autoantibodies. The presence of Raynaud's phenomenon, the severity of the xerostomia and dryness of the eyes are also more consistent with the primary form. In addition the patient has candidiasis which is the probable cause of the soreness.

TREATMENT

■ *How could you contribute to the management of this patient?*

Control of the underlying disease is not possible but the patient requires treatment for complications and continued follow up:
- Treat candidiasis and follow up regularly for recurrence.
- Preserve what salivary secretion remains; saliva is more effective than saliva substitutes.
  — Sip water rather than drinking it, so as to expand remaining saliva and not wash it from the mouth.
  — Whenever possible avoid drugs which cause xerostomia.
  — Maintain fluid intake.
  — Stimulate residual salivary flow using chewing gum (sugar-free).
  — Consider using pilocarpine in severe cases (though side-effects and an appropriate dosing regime can be problematic).
- Prevent and treat dental caries
  — Avoid sweets or overuse of citrus fruit to stimulate salivary flow.
  — Appropriate dietary analysis, preventive advice and fluoride treatment.
  — Treat caries.
- Consider using saliva substitutes though these are generally unsatisfactory and not liked by patients.
  — Carboxymethyl-cellulose and similar starch-based liquids.
  — Mucin-based preparations are more effective and generally better tolerated.

- Warn patient about, and follow up for, attacks of acute bacterial ascending sialadenitis which destroy residual gland function. Treat aggressively if it develops.
- Ensure continued ophthalmological follow up.
- Inform patient's general medical practitioner to ensure follow up for other complications. Involvement of other exocrine glands can lead to dry skin, dry vagina, pancreatic dysfunction and lung disease.
- Warn patient and follow up for development of persistent salivary gland swelling.
- Provide continued reassurance and care for patients with this distressing condition.

■ *What is the significance of the development of salivary gland swelling?*

This is usually the first sign of lymphoma development; 10% or more of patients with primary Sjögren's syndrome eventually develop lymphoma and in some cases it is the presenting sign. The lymphoma is usually a form of low grade B-cell lymphoma (MALT type) which has a slow indolent growth pattern, remains localized to the salivary glands for a long period and initially responds well to treatment. However, high grade lymphoma may also develop.

CASE

6

A lump on the gingiva

Summary

A 48-year-old man presents to you in general dental practice with a gingival swelling. What is the cause and what would you do?

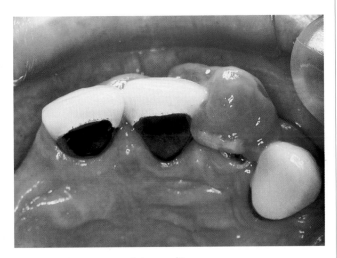

Fig. 6.1 Appearance of the swelling.

HISTORY

Complaint

The patient complains of a lump on the gum at the front of his mouth on the left side. It sometimes bleeds, usually after brushing or eating hard food but it is not painful.

History of complaint

The swelling has been present for 4 months and has grown slowly during this period. It was never painful but now looks unsightly. The patient gives no history of other mucosal or skin lesions.

Medical history

The patient has hypertension, controlled with atenolol 50 mg daily.

EXAMINATION

Extraoral examination

He is healthy-looking but slightly overweight. There are no palpable cervical lymph nodes.

Intraoral examination

The patient is partially dentate and has relatively few and extensively restored teeth. He wears an upper partial denture. The root of the upper lateral incisor is present and its carious surface lies at the level of the alveolar ridge. The teeth on each side of the lesion are restored with metal–ceramic crowns.

There is a mild degree of marginal gingivitis. Most of the interdental papillae are rounded and marginal inflammation is present around crowns. Flecks of subgingival calculus are visible.

■ *The appearance of the lesion is shown in Figure 6.1. Describe its features.*

Feature	Appearance
Site	Appears to arise from the gingival margin of the lateral incisor root or the interdental papilla mesially
Size	Approximately 10 × 7 mm
Shape and contour	Irregular rounded nodule. It is not possible to say whether it is pedunculated or sessile, though from its size and the fact that it overlies the lateral incisor root, it is probably pedunculated
Colour	Patchy red and pink with a thin grey translucent sheen. The surface is almost certainly ulcerated

If you were able to palpate the lesion you would find that it is fleshy and soft and attached by a thin base to the gingival margin. It bleeds readily from between the tooth and lesion when pressed with an instrument but it is not tender.

■ *From the information in the history and examination so far, what is your differential diagnosis?*

Likely:
— Pyogenic granuloma (if the patient had been female, pregnancy epulis would be considered)
— Fibrous epulis

Less likely:
— Peripheral giant cell granuloma
— Sinus papilla (parulis)

Unlikely:
— Papilloma
— Benign hamartoma or neoplasm
— Malignant neoplasm.

■ *Justify your differential diagnosis.*

A very wide range of lesions may affect the gingiva and many possible causes cannot be excluded on the basis of the information given so far. However, the gingiva is the site of predilection for a number of inflammatory hyperplastic lesions comprising fibrous tissue and epithelium. All are associated with poor oral hygiene and the lesion is almost certainly one of this type on statistical grounds.

Pyogenic granuloma is a localized proliferation of granulation tissue or very vascular fibrous tissue. It arises in association with a local irritant such as poor oral hygiene, calculus or the margin of a restoration. The present lesion has many features of the pyogenic granuloma: it is asymptomatic, soft and vascular, bleeds readily, and has an ulcerated surface. If the patient had been female, a pregnancy epulis, a variant of pyogenic granuloma arising during pregnancy would have been possible.

Fibrous epulis (gingival fibroepithelial polyp/nodule) is a nodule of more fibrous hyperplastic tissue. It is not usually ulcerated, is firmer on palpation and does not bleed so readily. Some fibrous epulides develop from pyogenic granulomas by maturation of the fibrous tissue and some arise de novo. They are usually associated with a local irritant in the same manner as pyogenic granulomas. The current lesion could well be a fibrous epulis, though its vascularity and red colour are more suggestive of pyogenic granuloma. These two names are really no more than convenient labels for lesions at opposite ends of a spectrum ranging from granulation tissue to dense fibrous tissue. All are hyperplastic.

The peripheral giant cell granuloma is another hyperplastic lesion which seems to develop in response to a local irritant. Clinically it may have a deep red maroon or blue colour, but is otherwise indistinguishable from pyogenic granuloma or fibrous epulis. However, histologically it is distinctive, containing numerous multinucleate osteoclast-like giant cells lying in a very cellular vascular stroma. The giant cell epulis is commoner in children, though it can arise in an adult. While it cannot be excluded, it is a less likely diagnosis for the present lesion.

Sinus papilla (parulis) is essentially a pyogenic granuloma developing at the opening of a sinus. Infection and inflammation are the stimuli inducing hyperplasia. If the sinus heals, the sinus papilla may disappear or it may mature into a small fibrous nodule. The usual site is on the alveolar mucosa and the lesion is usually no more than 4 or 5 mm across. This is an unlikely cause.

Papillomas are lesions of proliferating epithelium. Their exact cause is unknown though it is generally considered that some are caused by human papilloma virus infection. Others do not appear to contain virus and may be benign neoplasms. Papillomas may arise at any site in the oral cavity but are often seen at the gingival margin and lips. Sometimes patients have warts on their fingers as well. Papillomas usually have a white spiky or frond-covered surface or a smoother cauliflower-like surface and neither is seen in the present lesion. Papillomas do not bleed easily and this seems an unlikely diagnosis.

It would not be useful to list the many other possible causes, but a few groups of lesions might also be considered.

Hamartomas and benign neoplasms can arise at all sites. If this were such a lesion a haemangioma would be likely in view of the vascularity. A haemangioma could appear very similar to a pyogenic granuloma.

Odontogenic tumours can occasionally arise extraosseously in the gingiva but usually form uninflamed sessile nodules.

Malignant neoplasms occasionally present in the gingiva. Metastatic deposits are commoner than primary lesions and leukaemia is the most likely cause. Kaposi's sarcoma might also be considered in an HIV-positive individual. Both these lesions are vascular, may bleed on pressure and ulcerate.

FURTHER EXAMINATION AND INVESTIGATIONS

■ *What further examinations and investigations would you perform? Explain why.*

The definitive diagnosis will require a biopsy, and excision is indicated. However a number of other investigations (Table 6.1) need to be performed to identify possible causes. If the cause is left untreated the lesion may recur after excision.

The results of these further examinations are shown in Table 6.1.

DIFFERENTIAL DIAGNOSIS

■ *What is the most likely diagnosis?*

On the basis of the clinical appearance and the results of the tests in Table 6.1, the lesion is almost certainly a pyogenic granuloma or fibrous epulis.

TREATMENT

■ *What treatment would you provide?*

- Excision biopsy
- Removal of causative factors, i.e. plaque and calculus
- Provide treatment for the generalized periodontitis
- Extract or restore the lateral incisor root.

■ *Would you perform this biopsy in general dental practice? What complications might develop?*

Yes: this amounts to no more than the removal of a flap of gingiva, and ideally this would be performed in general practice. The only significant complication might be bleeding because this is a very vascular lesion. However, haemostasis should not prove a problem because pressure can be readily applied to the gingival margin.

■ *How would you obtain a report on the biopsy specimen?*

Most histopathology departments, either specialized oral pathology departments associated with dental schools, or departments in district general or other hospitals, provide postal or courier pathology services for the dentists and/or medical practitioners in their area.

The steps to be taken after removal are shown in Table 6.2.

Table 6.1 Investigations and findings

Test	Reason	Findings in this patient
Periodontal examination	To assess pocketing around the lesion and detect subgingival calculus, a common cause	There is generalized chronic adult periodontitis with loss of attachment of 3–4 mm. There is a 5-mm probing depth adjacent to the lesion, most of which is false pocket below the lesion. This pocket and others contain subgingival calculi
Tests of vitality of the adjacent incisor and canine	To determine whether the cause could be irritation from a periapical infection draining into the pocket	Both teeth are vital on electric pulp testing
Periapical view of the incisor and canine	Not useful for diagnosis but might be indicated on the basis of probing or vitality tests.	Not indicated

Table 6.2 Obtaining a report on a biopsy specimen

Aim	Procedure
Avoid distortion or crushing of specimen	If a suture has been placed through the lesion to hold it and prevent it being lost in the vacuum, do not remove it. Cut the thread a centimetre or so from the lesion.
Ensure rapid and efficient fixation	Place immediately in 10 times the tissue volume of 10% formol saline (available in biopsy containers from pharmacies, hospital suppliers and some pathology departments). In the absence of fixative, postpone the biopsy if possible. Spirits and other solutions used in dental surgeries are ineffective. An unfixed specimen will autolyse (rot) on the way to the laboratory.
Provide the pathologist with sufficient clinical information to enable diagnosis	Fill in a request form or write a letter including the patient's name, age and sex, a complete clinical description of the lesion, the differential diagnosis and medical history. Include any details of previous lesions or lesions elsewhere in the mouth. Do not forget your own name and practice address and phone number.
Protect those handling the specimen in transit	Package the specimen according to the Post Office regulations for sending hazardous materials through the post. Make sure the container is labelled with a hazard sticker identifying the contents as formalin. Place the specimen container in either an unbreakable second container or box with padding. Include enough absorbent material (e.g. tissue) to soak up all the formalin in the pack in the event of breakage. Label the package 'Pathology specimen – handle with care' and send by first-class post.

DIAGNOSIS

■ *The microscopic appearances of the biopsy specimen are shown in Figures 6.2 and 6.3. What do you see and how do you interpret them?*

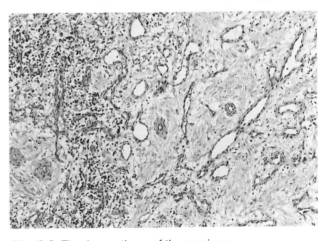

Fig. 6.3 The deeper tissue of the specimen.

The surface is ulcerated and covered by a slough of fibrin containing nuclei of inflammatory cells. At higher power you would be able to identify these as neutrophils. Below the surface is a pale-stained tissue in which the endothelial lining of numerous small blood vessels stands out. The vessels have a radiating pattern and point towards the surface reflecting a pattern of growth outwards from the centre. Between the vessels there is a little fibrin and the tissue is oedematous or myxoid or both. More deeply there is a cluster of inflammatory cells and collagen bundles are more prominent between the vessels.

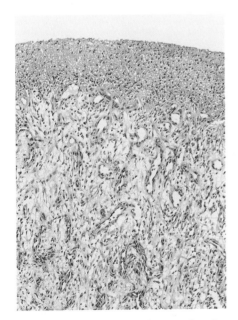

Fig. 6.2 Histological appearance of the surface layers of the excision specimen.

The lesion is a nodule of ulcerated maturing granulation and fibrous tissue.

■ *What is the diagnosis?*

Pyogenic granuloma.

ANOTHER POSSIBILITY

■ *Is a more conservative approach to treatment ever justified?*

Yes: elimination of the causative factors may induce considerable resolution. However, the degree of resolution varies; softer more vascular lesions shrink most and firmer more fibrous lesions hardly at all. Removal of calculus and improved oral hygiene may cause partial resolution and leave a smaller lesion which is easier to excise and bleeds much less. Such a course of action is often appropriate for treatment of pregnancy epulis, both because of the wish to avoid the procedure during pregnancy and because excision during pregnancy carries a risk of recurrence. Definitive excision may then be delayed until after parturition. Occasionally resolution is almost complete and no further treatment is required.

CASE 7 Pain on biting

Summary

A 32-year-old man presents at your general dental practice surgery with intermittent pain on biting. Identify the cause and discuss treatment options.

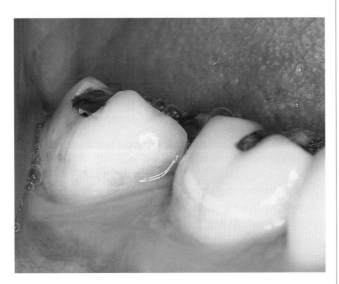

Fig. 7.1 The teeth in the lower right quadrant.

HISTORY

Complaint

He complains of pain on biting which is unpredictable, extremely painful and sharp but poorly localized. It originates in the lower right quadrant and lasts a very short time, only as long as the teeth are in contact, and is so painful that he has become accustomed to eating on the left. The pain only arises on biting hard foods or deliberately clenching his teeth. Apart from these sharp electric shock-like pains he has no other symptoms.

History of complaint

The pain is a recent phenomenon, having been first noticed a month or two ago. At first it was frequent but it has become less of a problem now that he has learnt to avoid triggering the pain. He has not noticed the pain being provoked by hot or cold.

Dental history

The patient has been a regular attender at your practice since childhood. He has a small number of relatively small restorations. At his last appointment, some 4 months ago you placed an amalgam restoration in the lower right second molar.

■ *Based on what you know already what are the likely causes? Explain why.*

A pulpal pain is the most likely cause because the pain appears to originate in a tooth and is poorly localized. Pain of periodontal ligament origin should be well localized. However, pulpitis appears not to be present because there is no sensitivity to hot or cold. Pulpitis caused by placement of the recent amalgams and pain due to caries or exposed dentine can be excluded for the same reasons.

A crack in the tooth or electrogalvanic pain are possible causes suggested by pain on biting. Both are triggered by tooth–tooth contact.

Trigeminal neuralgia should be considered as an unlikely nondental cause. It causes paroxysmal stabbing or electric shock-like facial pain in distributions of the trigeminal nerve and may be initiated by touching or moving trigger zones. It usually affects the middle-aged or elderly. The history of pain on biting is almost conclusive of a dental cause but it can be difficult to exclude trigeminal neuralgia in some patients, particularly when trigger zones lie in the mouth or attacks are triggered by eating. If no dental cause is found, the possibility of trigeminal neuralgia may need further investigation.

Acute periodontitis caused by an occlusal high spot on the recently placed amalgam needs to be considered. However, although this could cause great tenderness on biting it would be expected that the pain from the bruised periodontium would be present at other times. Also, such periodontally sensed pain would be well localized.

■ *What additional questions would you ask? Why?*

The patient should be asked about clenching or bruxing of the teeth because the additional occlusal load can cause fracture and will determine treatment options.

The patient describes a habit of nocturnal bruxism with some tenderness of masticatory muscles at times of stress.

EXAMINATION

Extraoral examination

There is a suspicion of hypertrophy of the masseter muscles on clenching.

Intraoral examination

The incisal edges of the upper and lower anterior teeth are worn and the dentine is exposed. The cusps of the posterior teeth are slightly flattened or rounded consistent with mild attrition. There is no evidence of any loss of attachment or gingival recession.

The appearances of the teeth in the lower right quadrant are shown in Figure 7.1. The lower right molars and premolars contain small- to moderate-sized MOD amalgam restorations, those in the molars having small buccal extensions. The upper molars have small separate MO and DO amalgams, the DO amalgams having buccal extensions. The upper premolars are unrestored.

■ **What features of the restorations would you note particularly?**

The restorations should be inspected for occlusal high spots, indicated by a burnished mark on the occlusal surface. Premature occlusal contact could be confirmed with articulating paper and relieving the area would cure the pain confirming the diagnosis.

Though they are unlikely causes for this particular pain, marginal caries, poor marginal adaptation or a cracked restoration should be sought.

DIFFERENTIAL DIAGNOSIS

■ **What is your differential diagnosis? Why?**

The pain is almost certainly caused by a cracked cusp or crown. The presence of masseteric hypertrophy and attrition on the occlusal surfaces of the teeth would suggest a parafunctional habit which could predispose the tooth to cracking.

Galvanic pain may be excluded because there are no occluding restorations of dissimilar metals.

■ **Which tooth would you suspect? Why?**

The lower second molar appears the most likely to be cracked. It should be investigated first because the pain seems to have started shortly after restoration.
The risk of cracking depends on the size of restorations. The upper teeth have small restorations which are limited to fissures and mesial and distal surfaces. In the upper molar the ridge of enamel joining the distobuccal to mesiopalatal cusps is intact so that cusps are unlikely to be undermined.

Intact teeth can also crack, though usually only in association with increased occlusal load. The most susceptible teeth are the premolars because moderately sized amalgams undermine the lingual and palatal cusps in the small crowns. Lower first molars are also prone to crack because they tend to contain the largest restorations in the mouth.

Root-filled teeth are prone to crack but obviously could not cause a pulpal pain. Symptoms are only produced when the periodontal ligament is involved and they are well localized.

INVESTIGATIONS

■ **What tests and further examinations would you perform to identify the causative tooth? What do the results tell you?**

The investigations are described in Table 7.1.

On performing these tests you discover that all the teeth in the quadrant are vital. Biting on cotton wool on the lower second molar provokes pain which the patient

Table 7.1 Identifying the causative tooth

Investigation	Significance
Tests of vitality of all teeth in the lower right quadrant should be performed, either with an electric pulp tester or a cold stimulus.	The pain must originate from a vital tooth. It is also possible that the cracked tooth might be hypersensitive. This could aid diagnosis though hypersensitivity to testing would not be expected in the absence of pain on hot and cold. Vitality might also affect the choice of treatment.
Close examination with a good light (a bright fibre optic is especially useful for transillumination). A soluble dye such as a disclosing agent may be painted onto the crown. After the excess is washed off small amounts may remain in the crack rendering it visible.	May reveal a crack.
Attempts to stimulate the pain by pressing the handle of an instrument against each cusp, preferably from more than one direction.	Pain indicates a cracked cusp and the causative cusp is identified.
Ask the patient to bite hard on a soft object such as a cotton wool roll.	This transmits pressure to the whole occlusal surface and forces the cusps slightly apart. Pain on biting suggests a cracked tooth.
Place a wooden wedge against each cusp in turn and ask the patient to bite on each.	This is a more selective test to identify the cusp or cusps which are cracked. By placing the wedge on different surfaces of the cusp it may be possible to tell in which direction the crack runs. There may be pain on biting but pain which is worse on release of pressure is said to be characteristic.
Radiograph	To exclude the possibility of caries and to assess the feasibility of root filling the tooth should it be necessary. The radiograph is unlikely to be of direct help in diagnosis and might not be necessary if other investigations successfully identify the cracked cusp.

Table 7.2 Restoration options for cracked teeth

Option	Advantages and disadvantages
No treatment	This is not an option, even if the patient is happy to put up with the pain. Cracks may propagate into the pulp, allow bacterial contamination and devitalize the tooth.
Removal of the cracked portion followed by restoration	This is unsafe. Levering of the cracked portion risks a catastrophic fracture with pulpal communication. Many cracks are incomplete and leverage may propagate them in unpredictable directions. Just occasionally the fragment will be limited to enamel and dentine of the crown, particularly where the tooth already contains a large restoration undermining the cusp, but even then a deliberate fracture is not recommended.
Full or partial coverage gold indirect restoration	This is the treatment of choice. The preparation should finish supragingivally wherever possible. Gold is malleable and allows some plastic deformation which is not possible with ceramics or composites which are more brittle. Full occlusal coverage is needed to protect the tooth from further damage and a casting can provide some splinting, reducing the potential for further cracks.
Full coverage bonded porcelain crown	Full coverage with porcelain bonded to metal has the advantage of a better appearance but the ceramic is brittle. This disadvantage may be offset by using an adhesive to lute the crown. There is then the potential for the crack to be sealed by the infiltrating cement.
Adhesive restoration	In theory an adhesive restoration would cement the crack together and prevent movement of the two fragments. However, on curing, adhesive materials undergo polymerization shrinkage which places further stress on the crack and may propagate it further.
Porcelain inlay/onlay	These suffer the same disadvantages of metal fused to porcelain crowns.

identifies as the same as that on biting. No particular cusp can be identified and no crack can be found.

TREATMENT

■ *What would you do next? Explain why.*

The path of the crack must be defined as far as possible because this will determine treatment options. The restoration(s) in the tooth should be removed and a further attempt made to find the crack using transillumination and dye as described above. If the crack appears to enter the pulp or be directed towards it, root treatment will be required.

After investigation the crack is found to run across the mesiolingual cusp and disappear subgingivally. It does not appear to enter the pulp.

■ *What are the treatment options for restoring cracked teeth? What are their advantages and disadvantages?*

These are listed in Table 7.2.

■ *If the cracked portion had already been broken off at presentation and the pulp were not involved, what restoration options would have been open to you?*

Assuming no second crack were present, this would present a simple choice. One of the methods described above could be used and this would have the advantage that further cracks would be prevented. In view of the history of bruxism this might be an appropriate option.

However, most cracks are single and it would also be possible to adopt a more conservative approach and restore with a composite and a dentine bonding agent or a sandwich restoration. The latter uses a glass ionomer to replace the

dentine and a composite to replace the enamel. An amalgam restoration is also simple and highly effective. Both these would require the cusp to be reduced in height to reduce the occlusal load.

■ *Suppose you had been unable to identify the causative tooth using the methods described above. What would you try next?*

Sometimes it is difficult to identify a crack. The pain is poorly localized and a first step would be to repeat the whole procedure on the upper molars and premolars in case the patient has incorrectly localized the pain.

If no crack is identified, the restorations must be removed from any further teeth which appear to be likely causes. Finally, the most suspect tooth may have a tight fitting copper band or orthodontic band cemented around it. This can be left in position for several weeks to see whether the pain is abolished, and is a particularly useful test when the pain is felt infrequently.

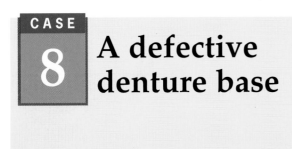

CASE 8

A defective denture base

Summary

The acrylic denture base and chrome–cobalt casting shown both have defects caused by similar mechanisms. Can you identify the problem and its causes, which are different in the two examples.

ACRYLIC COMPLETE DENTURE

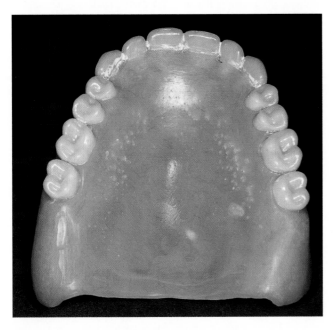

Fig. 8.1 The heat-processed 'acrylic', poly(methylmethacrylate) denture base.

■ *A heat-processed 'acrylic', poly(methylmethacrylate) denture base is shown in Figure 8.1. What do you see and how do you interpret these observations?*

The denture base has a cluster of small round holes in a horseshoe-shaped distribution just inside the teeth. The defects are more frequent in areas of thicker acrylic. Each defect appears to be round, some are completely enclosed in acrylic, while others communicate with the surface via sharply defined holes.

The presence of numerous small holes or defects within the acrylic is known as porosity.

■ *What are the types of porosity? How do they manifest and what are their causes?*

The types of porosity are presented in Table 8.1.

This denture has suffered from gaseous porosity and the appearances are typical but more extensive than usually seen.

■ *What causes monomer to vaporize during processing?*

The boiling point of methylmethacrylate is 100.3°C at standard temperature and pressure. If the boiling point is exceeded then the methylmethacrylate vaporizes and bubbles produce porous defects. The polymerization of methylmethacrylate is exothermic and will contribute to vaporization if precautions are not taken to reduce the temperature. Because the process is heat-dependent, it is most likely to develop in thick sections of the denture and in the last portions to be polymerized.

■ *How is gaseous porosity normally prevented?*

Methylmethacrylate should be polymerized at a low temperature and under pressure. Packing the dough under pressure raises the boiling point of the methylmethacrylate, and polymerization at 72°C for 16 hours (or 72°C for 2 hours and 100°C for a further 2 hours) followed by slow cooling gives time for the heat of the exothermic reaction to dissipate.

Table 8.1 Types of porosity

Defect	Manifestation	Cause
Contraction porosity	Porosity throughout the denture. The denture may be the incorrect shape.	Insufficient material packed into the flask, or inadequate flasking pressure. Correct use of the trial packing stage should eliminate this.
Gaseous porosity	Porosity in a localized area of the denture base, particularly in the thicker parts. Each defect is round and sharply defined.	Vaporization of monomer during processing.
Granular porosity	Porosity appears in thin sections of the denture, which often have a 'white and frosty' appearance.	Incorrect polymer:monomer ratio when producing the dough, or failing to pack the flask at the dough stage.

CHROME–COBALT CASTING

■ *A chrome–cobalt denture framework is shown in Figure 8.2. What do you see and how do you interpret these changes?*

The metal has numerous small perforating holes. They are of various sizes and some have coalesced to form large defects.

■ *What are the common defects in chrome–cobalt castings? How may they be prevented?*

See Table 8.2.

■ *Which of these defects affects the present casting? Explain why.*

The casting defects are small and round, like those in the acrylic denture, and also appear to be caused by gas bubble formation. This is another example of porosity but it is much more extensive than is seen when the investment is too thick or gas dissolves in the alloy. In this case a more fundamental mistake must have been made and the cause is probably use of the wrong investment material.

If a framework is invested in a gypsum-bonded investment, the investment will break down at a lower temperature than

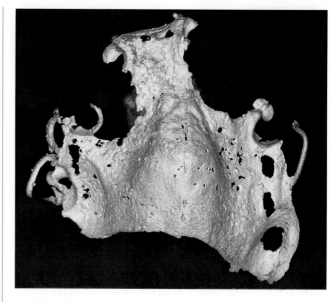

Fig. 8.2 The cobalt–chromium partial denture casting.

the melting point of the alloy. The $CaSO_4$ binder reacts with the SiO_2 refractory to produce SO_3 gas, bubbles of which cause porosity in the casting. Gypsum-bonded investments are used for gold-based alloys and phosphate-bonded investments must be used for Co–Cr based alloys.

Table 8.2 Common defects in chrome–cobalt castings

Defect	Cause	Preventive measure
Porosity: spherical voids	Investment too thick	Use the correct powder:liquid ratio
	Gases dissolve in the alloy and form bubbles on cooling	Do not overheat the alloy
Porosity: irregular voids	Casting shrinkage	Ensure sprues are of the correct diameter
	Turbulent flow of the alloy	Ensure sprues are in the correct position
Incomplete cast: rounded margins	Back pressure of air in the mould	Use a porous investment or include vents
Incomplete cast: short casting	Insufficient alloy	Use sufficient alloy
	Mould too cold when cast	Ensure the correct operating temperature
	Insufficient casting force	Ensure the machine is correctly set up
Fins	Investment cracking	Use the correct investment and do not heat too rapidly
Rough surface	Investment breakdown	Use the correct investment and do not overheat
	Air bubbles on wax pattern	Use a wetting agent
Distortion	Stress relief of the wax pattern	Warm the wax thoroughly before making the pattern
Cast too small	Insufficient investment expansion	Use the correct operating temperature
Cast too large	Too much investment expansion	Use the correct investment for the alloy, and the correct operating temperature

Sudden collapse

Summary

A 55-year-old male patient suddenly collapses in your general dental practice. What is the cause and what would you do?

HISTORY

Complaint

The patient has attended for a routine dental appointment to receive some simple conservation work under local anaesthetic. He is a regular attender but dislikes injections.

Twenty minutes after injection of the local anaesthetic he suddenly becomes anxious and complains of a pain in his chest. He is breathless. When your nurse asks the patient if he is OK there is no response.

Medical history

Having checked the medical history just before starting treatment you are aware that the patient is a well-controlled insulin-dependent diabetic. He suffers hypertension and takes enalapril 20 mg daily (Innovace) and is overweight. He smokes 20 cigarettes a day and describes himself as a 'social drinker', consuming 30 units of alcohol each week.

■ *What would you do immediately?*

Check to see whether the patient is conscious. Make a determined effort to rouse him by shaking him and asking loudly whether he can hear you.

The patient does not respond.

■ *What causes of sudden loss of consciousness might affect a patient undergoing dental treatment?*

The important causes of unexpected loss of consciousness are:
• vasovagal attack (faint)
• hypoglycaemia
• cardiac arrest
• steroid crisis
Loss of consciousness may also follow several other emergencies including respiratory obstruction or respiratory failure, epilepsy, stroke or anaphylactic shock, in which the cause is likely to be evident.

■ *How may these causes of loss of consciousness be differentiated?*

Cause	Signs and symptoms
Vasovagal attack (faint)	Often associated with anxiety. Usually, though not always, some premonitory symptoms of faintness before losing consciousness. Cold clammy skin, pallor, initially bradycardia and low pulse volume followed by tachycardia and a full pulse. Rapid recovery on placing supine or slightly head down (maximum recommended inclination 10°).
Hypoglycaemia	Seen in starved patients or diabetics with relative insulin overdose caused by starvation or stress. Rapid recovery on administering oral glucose or, if unconscious, glucagon followed by oral glucose on regaining consciousness.
Steroid crisis	Seen only in those taking systemic steroids in relative insufficiency as a result of stress.
Cardiac arrest	No central pulse. Usually history of angina, coronary arterial disease, hypertension or other risk factor.

■ *Which is the most likely cause in this case? Why?*

In this case the cause is very likely to be cardiac arrest. The symptom of pain in the chest radiating to the neck and arm is characteristic of myocardial infarction, the commonest cause of cardiac arrest, and is not seen in the other causes of collapse. Diabetes, hypertension and a high alcohol intake are all risk factors for atheromatous arterial disease and its complication of myocardial infarction.

■ *Does cardiac arrest always follow myocardial infarction?*

No. The heart may continue to pump unless a large area of the myocardium or conducting tissue is damaged. Cardiac arrest may also follow hypoxia or respiratory obstruction.

■ *How will you confirm your provisional diagnosis?*

For a diagnosis of cardiac arrest, the patient must:
• have no central pulse (carotid or femoral)
• be unconscious.

EXAMINATION

You place a hand on the patient's neck to feel the carotid pulse. He feels cold and clammy. Even though it is only half a minute since he lost consciousness the patient already looks grey and he is beginning to look cyanosed. You cannot detect any carotid pulse.

■ *What is the current protocol for assessing and managing sudden collapse (assuming you are the only person present)?*

It is critically important to start Basic Life Support (BLS) procedures immediately without further consideration of possible causes. The current (June 1998) Resuscitation Council guidelines for the management of cardiac arrest are:

1. Check area for danger.

2. Assess responsiveness by shaking and shouting.

3. Call for help from those around you.

4. Open the airway (tilt head back and chin lift or jaw thrust).

5. Check mouth for vomit/debris and remove with finger sweeps.

6. Assess breathing
   — listen and feel for breathing whilst observing chest movements (up to 10 seconds).
   — If NO breathing, phone for help immediately ('999') then:

7. Give two slow ventilations (up to 5 attempts)

8. Assess carotid pulse (up to 10 seconds)
   — If pulse present but still NOT breathing: give 10 ventilations and re-check carotid pulse every minute.
   — If NO pulse present then:

9. Perform 15 chest compressions of 4–5 cm each on the lower third of the sternum at a rate of 100 per minute, followed by 2 ventilations

10. If the pulse is restored, reassess breathing and if satisfactory place the patient in the recovery position and administer oxygen. Otherwise, continue ventilations and compressions until help arrives.

■ *What are Basic and Advanced Life Support?*

Basic Life Support (BLS) is the diagnosis and immediate management of cardiac arrest (of whatever aetiology) without the use of equipment. It is intended to be performed by both lay and professional personnel in any location. It represents the absolute minimum standard of resuscitation skills which all dentists, dental hygienists and dental nurses must acquire and maintain.

Advanced Life Support (ALS) is concerned with the restoration of spontaneous circulation and stabilization of the cardiovascular system. Techniques include ECG assessment, defibrillation and the administration of drugs. ALS should be available in practices administering general anaesthesia or advanced (multidrug) sedation techniques.

■ *What is the aim of Basic Life Support?*

To protect the brain from irreversible hypoxic damage. This develops within 3–4 minutes of cardiac arrest in a previously healthy and well-oxygenated individual. Basic Life Support delays the rate of deterioration of cerebral function and maximizes the chances of ALS being successful. Effective BLS followed by prompt ALS and hospital admission greatly increases the patient's chance of survival.

■ *Why not dial '999' as soon as the patient loses consciousness?*

The most common cause of sudden loss of consciousness in the dental chair is a vasovagal attack (faint) which does not require attendance by the emergency services. The call for help in step 3 is intended to summon local helpers such as dental nurses or receptionist.

■ *What is the most common cause of failure or difficulty with BLS?*

Airway obstruction in the unconscious patient is the commonest problem and is usually due to the relaxed tongue falling back to obliterate the airway in the oropharynx. This may be overcome by measures which pull the tongue forward such as head tilt (neck lift), chin lift and jaw thrust. Blood, vomit or other foreign materials (including poorly fitting or broken dentures) may also obstruct the airway.

■ *Should dentures be removed during BLS?*

Only if they are loose or broken. Well-fitting dentures usually facilitate a good oral seal during expired air (mouth-to-mouth) ventilation.

■ *If the patient is not breathing (step 6), can you be certain that the patient has suffered cardiac arrest?*

No. The diagnosis depends upon loss of consciousness and *absence of a central pulse*. However, calling 999 for professional assistance if there is respiratory arrest at this point is sensible, because cardiac arrest follows respiratory arrest very quickly.

■ *Having dialled 999, what information should your helper give the operator?*

- your name
- address (with directions)
- your telephone number
- that a patient has collapsed with a suspected cardiac arrest.

Although this sounds simple, hurried calls may omit essential information. Response to cardiac arrest is usually provided at highest priority by a specialized team and is not a routine ambulance call. Failure to provide your telephone number leaves the emergency services unable to return your call.

■ *The table describes BLS provided by one person. If there were two trained staff to deal with the emergency how would the procedure differ?*

The ratio of ventilations to compressions would be changed to 1:5 but all other parameters remain the same.

PROGNOSIS

■ *Is it likely that your patient will recover spontaneously?*

Unfortunately not. Even with prompt ALS support from a specialist team the chances of death are greater than 50%. This may seem a poor chance of survival but if BLS and ALS are delayed, less than 2% of patients will live. In this case the patient recovered following ALS care provided by a specialist ambulance team who arrived at the practice 12 minutes after the 999 call was placed; a very rapid response.

■ *How long would you continue to provide BLS?*

Until help arrives or you are exhausted.

■ *How can you increase your chances of providing effective Basic Life Support?*

Only by regular practical instruction and testing the competence of yourself and your practice team. BLS cannot be learned from a book.

Pain after extraction

Summary

A 34-year-old lady presents with severe pain a few days after tooth extraction. What is the cause and what can be done?

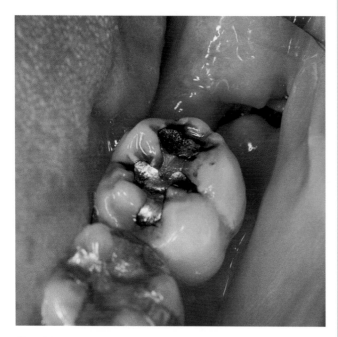

Fig. 10.1 The appearance of the socket.

HISTORY

Complaint

She complains of a distressingly severe pain from an extraction socket in the left side of her mandible. The pain is localized to the extraction socket and is not sensitive to hot or cold. It is a constant, dull boring pain unrelieved by aspirin or paracetamol preparations. It prevents the patient performing any normal activity and kept her awake last night.

History of complaint

The patient underwent surgical removal of the lower left third molar tooth at her dentist 4 days ago. The extraction had proved more difficult than expected and involved repeated attempted elevation and a small amount of bone removal using a bur. Following the extraction, bleeding stopped normally. The extraction

site had been tender but apparently was healing slowly until the pain started yesterday. Since then she has also noticed halitosis and a bad taste.

Medical history

The patient is otherwise fit and well. She is taking an oral contraceptive and no other positive findings were revealed by the medical history.

EXAMINATION

Extraoral examination

The patient has moderate extraoral swelling of the facial soft tissues overlying the extraction socket and some early discoloration of the skin by ecchymosis. There is trismus and she is able to open her mouth to only 22 mm interincisal clearance. There are no palpable lymph nodes in the deep cervical chain or submandibular triangle.

Intraoral examination

Halitosis is noticeable. The appearance of the socket is shown in Figure 10.1. The lower left third molar socket contains no tissue, only food debris. The surrounding soft tissues are slightly swollen but not significantly inflamed as judged by redness.

DIAGNOSIS

■ *Based on what you know already, what is the most likely diagnosis?*

The diagnosis is most likely to be a dry socket (alveolar osteitis). The history of severe and persistent pain localized to the tooth socket appearing 3–5 days after extraction, particularly a traumatic one, is characteristic. The lack of local inflammation or enlarged lymph nodes is compatible with this diagnosis and argues against post-extraction infection either in the bone or soft tissue.

The diagnosis is confirmed by the examination which shows that the blood clot has been lost from the socket. In severe cases the bone of the socket may be exposed, though this does not appear to be so in this patient.

Halitosis is the result of food debris in the socket being degraded by a partially anaerobic bacterial flora. The trismus is almost certainly related to the surgical trauma of extraction.

■ *What other causes of post-extraction pain are there? Are they likely in this case?*

Pain from surgical trauma to tissues should be considered when extraction is difficult. However pain starts immediately after sensation is regained in the area and responds to analgesics. Tenderness is characteristic, rather than spontaneous pain.

Osteomyelitis is rare but should be considered because of its severity and difficulty of treatment, especially if diagnosed late. It causes a deep boring pain, not dissimilar from dry socket, but is poorly localized. Osteomyelitis is almost exclusively seen in patients who are immunocompromised or have sclerosis of the bone of the jaws. It usually takes several weeks to become evident.

Fractured mandible is a very rare complication of extraction. It might be considered if swelling and bruising appear out of proportion to dental extraction. However it is usually evident clinically if the fracture is displaced.

Retained root fragments are surprisingly rarely a cause of long-term pain, though the surgical trauma of the failed extraction may cause pain. Root fragments are almost never found in a dry socket.

None of these alternative causes match the patient's symptoms or signs as well as dry socket.

■ *What investigations would you carry out?*

At this stage, the history and examination are completely compatible with the diagnosis and no investigations are indicated. If there were features of infection, culture of pus and antibiotic sensitivity would be necessary and the temperature should be taken. Radiographs are not useful unless a root fragment is suspected but cannot be seen or palpated. Even if osteomyelitis is suspected, radiographs would not provide useful information because there has been insufficient time for the characteristic radiographic changes to develop.

■ *What is a dry socket?*

A dry socket is one from which the blood clot is lost before it can become stabilized by ingrowth of granulation tissue. The exposed bone surface becomes colonized by anaerobic bacteria and spirochaetes and is partially and superficially devitalized. Loss of blood clot is thought to be the result of excessive fibrinolysis caused by bacterial, local tissue or salivary factors.

In the absence of a blood clot, healing is delayed because soft tissue must grow from the gingival margin to cover the bone and fill the socket.

■ *What factors predispose to dry socket?*

The risk factors associated with development of dry socket are:

Surgical or traumatic extraction

Mandibular extraction, especially third molar

Female patient, especially if on contraceptive medication

Patient who smokes

Infection or recent infection at site

Periodontal disease or acute necrotizing ulcerative gingivitis elsewhere in the mouth

Local bone disease or sclerosis reducing blood supply for clot formation, as in Paget's disease, cemento-osseous dysplasia and after radiotherapy

Excessive use of local anaesthetic; vasoconstrictor in excess around the socket may prevent formation of blood clot

History of previous dry socket

Young adult to middle-aged patient

■ *How would you treat this patient?*

Reassure the patient that though extremely painful this condition does not signify any serious consequence of the extraction. Inform her that the socket will heal normally but more slowly than usual, and that during the healing period treatment can be provided to relieve the pain though she may have to return for several treatments.

Local treatment to the socket is the most effective measure. Irrigate the socket gently with warm saline or 0.12% chlorhexidine to remove the debris. Place a dressing into the mouth of the socket to prevent impaction of further food. Many proprietary dressings are available, including resorbable materials, antiseptic preparations and analgesic formulations. In practice almost all are satisfactory provided they are used appropriately and replaced as required. Care should be taken not to pack the socket full of the dressing because this would prevent it from filling up with granulation tissue as healing progresses.

Effective socket cleansing and socket hygiene are more important than the type of dressing used and the patient should be recalled every 2 days for retreatment if necessary. In severe cases a daily dressing may be appropriate initially, and as the socket heals and pain reduces the period between dressing may be extended. The trismus should be monitored and should reduce.

■ *What drugs might you prescribe?*

Antibiotics should not be prescribed because they are ineffective. Analgesics are also largely ineffective in the absence of local measures. A nonsteroidal anti-inflammatory drug should be adequate for most cases. The pain of dry socket has a reputation for severity and in the past controlled drugs have been prescribed. This is only occasionally justified but may need to be considered.

■ *How quickly will the pain be relieved?*

Improvement of symptoms will usually be noted within minutes or up to an hour, and more quickly if the dressing contains a local anaesthetic agent. Pain will start again a day or two after dressing, gradually increasing in severity. After a few days the pain will reduce and re-dressing may not be necessary. After about 10 days the socket should be filled with tissue and it will probably be asymptomatic for the last few days of healing.

■ *What if the condition persists for more than this or appears to be worsening?*

Failure to resolve in the longer term usually indicates the presence of small sequestra of devitalized lamina dura or root fragments. These are a normal sequela of extraction and are usually resorbed in the remodelling process during healing. Larger pieces may delay healing and sometimes sequestrate through the alveolar ridge mucosa many weeks after extraction, though they are not usually associated with significant pain. Periapical radiographs should be taken because only these have the resolution required to see the small sequestra, which may be less than half a millimetre in size. Occasionally, larger sequestra of lamina dura may be seen to be separating radiographically. If these are associated with symptoms and are not shed, surgical removal may become necessary. In practice this intervention is extremely rarely required, and sequestra are usually small and lost without being noticed.

The diagnosis will have to be reviewed and radiographs are also useful to exclude other causes for the pain. In the event that the nature of the pain has changed, or if the patient suffers any condition predisposing to osteomyelitis (local bone sclerosis, pathological or therapeutic immunosuppression), this possibility should be thoroughly investigated.

CASE 11

A loose tooth

Summary

A 25-year-old man presents in your general dental practice with a loose tooth. Identify the cause and summarize the treatment options.

Complaint

The patient complains of a loose tooth and points to his upper left lateral incisor which is crowned. He says it is uncomfortable when it moves and has become so mobile that he thinks it may fall out.

History of complaint

He has noticed that the tooth has become progressively looser over the last few months and would like a replacement. There has been no pain associated with the tooth but he is aware of an unpleasant taste which appears to emanate intermittently from his upper front teeth.

Dental history

The patient had been a regular attender at another dental practice for many years until he moved to your area. He is motivated and does not wish to lose any teeth.

Four years previously, the lateral and central incisors had been fractured in an accident at work. Both teeth sustained class II coronal fractures but were initially left untreated. Several months later another dental practitioner provided some restorations on both teeth and shortly afterwards the patient asked for the lateral incisor to be crowned because he was unhappy with the appearance.

Medical history

The patient has insulin-controlled diabetes. Otherwise he is fit and well and is taking no medication.

EXAMINATION

Extraoral examination

No submandibular or cervical lymph nodes are palpable.

Intraoral examination

The patient has an extensively restored dentition with a crowned upper left lateral incisor which is grade II mobile buccolingually but not vertically. There is generalized but mild redness and delayed bleeding on probing around the gingival margin associated with a small amount of plaque at the crown margin. However, there is no increase in probing depth around this tooth. There is no evidence of caries on any teeth and generally the periodontal condition is good. The adjacent teeth are firm. No sinuses are present to explain the bad taste and no pus is detected on periodontal probing.

■ *What additional questions might you ask?*

Did you notice the mobility suddenly increase or hear a crack from the tooth? The marked mobility without evidence of periodontitis suggests a root fracture.

The patient has noticed no sudden increase in mobility.

■ *How would you clinically assess the possibility of root fracture?*

By determining the axis of rotation of the mobile crown. Apply pressure forwards and backwards to identify how far down the root the axis of rotation appears to be.

When you do this you find that the crown appears to rotate about a point 2–3 mm below the gingival margin.

If rocking the crown produces bubbles of saliva at the gingival margin this would be an indicator of a root fracture communicating with a periodontal pocket or the gingival crevice. No such bubbles were seen.

■ *Based on what you know so far, what are the likely causes?*

Having excluded mobility caused by periodontitis and coronal bone loss, the two possibilities which remain the most likely are resorption or root fracture. The mobile tooth is rotating about a point just below the gingival margin so either process must affect the coronal part of the root.

Resorption of the apical half of the root would move the axis of rotation of the remaining tooth coronally. There would have to be extensive resorption to cause this degree of mobility and raise the axis of rotation so far. Resorption is a recognized complication of trauma to teeth and so this would be the most likely cause.

Root fracture is possible. No fracture was noted but the marked mobility would be consistent with a root fracture of the coronal part of the root. If there is a root fracture it would appear to be independent of the original trauma. Teeth which suffer coronal fractures do not usually suffer root fractures as well because the energy of the blow is transmitted less to the root. However, if a root fracture had been present for the last 4 years it might have triggered slow resorption, combining both possible causative factors.

An unsuspected lesion has destroyed the bone and/or the tooth root apically, leaving support only coronally; this is a remote possibility. The tooth would then be mobile about the remaining intact periodontal ligament. The commonest lesion to do this would be a radicular cyst arising on a nonvital tooth.

Table 11.1 Investigations to be carried out

Test	Reason	Problems
Vitality test	To check the vitality of all four upper and lower incisors and canines (excluding any known root filled teeth). Late loss of vitality is a complication of trauma and any one of these teeth could have periapical infection and be the cause of the bad taste. The vitality of the lateral incisor needs to be known, to plan treatment once the diagnosis is established.	Electric pulp tests are notoriously difficult to perform on crowned teeth and the results must be interpreted with caution. The lateral incisor has a metal ceramic bonded crown and the ceramic will insulate the tooth while the metal layer will diffuse the applied voltage and conduct the stimulus to the gingiva. The patient may mistake a gingival sensation for a vitality response.
Periapical radiograph	To detect the possible causes and assess bone levels around the teeth. To determine the pulp canal morphology in case root canal treatment is required, and the root morphology in case extraction is necessary.	Root fractures may be difficult to identify if the fragments are not separated. A second view at a slightly different angle may allow detection of a root fracture invisible in the first. However, this tooth is so mobile that any root fracture should be readily identified.

However this seems most unlikely as there is no expansion and the adjacent teeth are not displaced or mobile. A different lesion remains a remote possibility.

INVESTIGATIONS

■ *What investigations would you carry out? Why? What are the potential problems?*

See Table 11.1.

On performing the tests of tooth vitality you find that it is impossible to obtain a response from the upper left central and lateral incisors. All other anterior teeth appear vital.

■ *The periapical radiograph is shown in Figure 11.1. What do you see?*

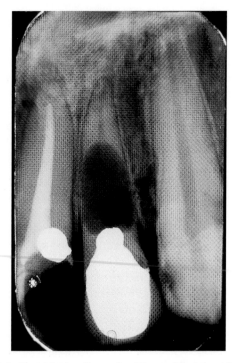

Fig. 11.1 Periapical radiograph of the mobile lateral incisor.

The left lateral incisor is crowned but not root filled. A large oval radiolucency fills the middle third of the root and extends laterally to replace the full width of the root and communicate with the periodontal ligament. The margins of the defect are smooth and sharply defined. The lamina dura around the apex appears intact. The bone level mesially and distally is coronal to the defect and there is no evidence of either horizontal or vertical bone loss. Very little root dentine remains below the crown and gingival margin.

The upper left central incisor is root filled. The filling appears well condensed and extends very close to the ideal level. The root appears to have a curve at the apex. There is a poorly defined radiolucency around the apex, mostly on its mesial side, where the lamina dura is missing.

The canine has mesial caries and its apical lamina dura is indistinct. However no obvious apical radiolucency is present.

■ *What is wrong with the radiograph in Figure 11.1?*

A regular pattern is superimposed over the whole film. This is a developing artefact caused by some film processors (e.g. Velopex) which use woven nylon bands to transport the film between solutions. If these bands are dirty or worn their surface texture transfers an imprint onto the film. A less marked example of the same artefact is shown in Figure 23.3.

Another uniform artefactual pattern results from exposing the wrong side of an intraoral film packet to the beam. The embossed metal backing foil casts a patterned shadow onto the film and the shielding causes an additional underexposure, differentiating this artefact from the one illustrated.

DIAGNOSIS

■ *What is your diagnosis?*

There is extensive internal resorption of the lateral incisor. The central incisor has a failed root filling with a periapical granuloma or abscess. The cause of the bad taste could be either intermittent drainage of pus from this periapical lesion or plaque trapped in the resorption defect or caries on the mesial surface of the upper left canine.

■ *What types of resorption are there? What are their characteristic features?*

Resorption is the process of removal of dental hard tissues by osteoclasts. There is usually some form of repair, either by reactionary dentine or bone, and repair may lead to ankylosis. All resorption is identical in its basic process, but it is convenient to subdivide resorption into clinically relevant types. Resorption may be classified as inflammatory or replacement types, or alternatively as internal or external types. All types may be transient or progressive.

Inflammatory resorption is associated with detectable inflammation and may be internal or external (apical or cervical). Inflammation may be evident radiographically, as radiolucency in the adjacent bone, or clinically as redness. The inflammatory type of resorption has the positive aspect that treatment of the cause of the inflammation may halt the resorption. Unfortunately this is not entirely predictable. Many cases of so-called inflammatory resorption, both internal and external, are not associated with significant inflammation clinically or histologically and are perhaps better regarded as idiopathic.

Replacement resorption is resorption accompanied by progressive replacement of the tooth by bone. It is often associated with ankylosis and is a complication of luxation injuries, particularly intrusion and avulsion. Inflammation is absent, so that treatment, which is difficult, must be directed at the resorption itself.

Internal resorption starts on the pulpal aspect of the dentine. It typically affects the middle third of the root and forms a well-demarcated defect with a smooth symmetrical shape. Internal resorption indicates that the pulp is vital and that, provided the lesion has not perforated the root, the process will be halted by root canal treatment.

External resorption starts on the outer surface of the tooth, usually on the root but occasionally on the crown in unerupted teeth. A microscopic degree of superficial external root resorption is normal and is usually repaired by cementum. Greater apical resorption may be seen radiographically on teeth which have been moved orthodontically. Extensive apical resorption may accompany periapical inflammation or infection on nonvital teeth. A nonvital pulp may also trigger external resorption of the root coronally by producing noxious products which diffuse outwards to the periodontal ligament along the dentinal tubules. Cervical resorption usually starts just below the gingival margin and may affect one or many teeth. Radiographically, the early stages may mimic the appearance of an infra bony periodontal pocket. All types of external resorption are irregular in outline and extensive lesions often spare a thin layer of dentine around the pulp so that the pulp can remain vital until a late stage.

■ *What causes resorption?*

Resorption and repair are physiological processes on the external surface of the root. On the pulpal surface resorption is pathological but repair is one of the pulp's responses to injury. External resorption is known to follow damage to the cementum layer or loss of vitality of cementum and this is thought to be why avulsion injury is so commonly followed by resorption. Cervical resorption is assumed to be primarily inflammatory in aetiology, caused by the periodontal flora, though this does not explain cases where multiple lesions affect several teeth.

Internal resorption must follow loss of the pre-dentine layer separating pulp from dentine, but the causes of this loss are unknown. A degree of inflammation or increased pulpal pressure are probably factors.

■ *What are the features of resorption?*

- Asymptomatic (unless an inflammatory cause is symptomatic).
- Internal resorption is only active in vital or partially vital teeth.
- External resorption may develop on vital or nonvital teeth.
- Resorption itself does not compromise vitality until the pulp communicates with the mouth.
- Usually slow and intermittent, occasionally very rapid.
- Mobility or pathological fracture.
- 'Pink spot': pulp visible through the crown.
- Ankylosis (continuity of tooth and bone).
- Radiolucency and loss of tooth substance.

■ *What are the signs of ankylosis?*

- Lack of normal mobility
- High pitched metallic percussive sound
- Infra occlusion (in the growing jaw)
- Sometimes identifiable radiographically as a bridged periodontal ligament
- Patchy 'moth-eaten' root surface/lamina dura.

■ *What is your diagnosis?*

Internal resorption, probably as a late sequela of the previous trauma or restoration of the teeth. Resorption is advanced and the root has suffered a pathological fracture making the coronal fragment very mobile.

The upper central incisor has a persistent periapical periodontitis despite root canal treatment.

TREATMENT

■ *How would you manage this problem in the short and long term?*

The prognosis for the lateral incisor is poor and it requires extraction. It cannot be restored because the resorption has involved the periodontal ligament around much of the tooth circumference. A tooth with a more localized perforation might be repaired surgically. However, in combination with the necessary root canal treatment, this would be heroic treatment with an unpredictable chance of success. Repair is more likely to be practical for external cervical resorption.

Time must be given for alveolar remodelling before the definitive restoration is made and a temporary replacement will be required.

■ *What are your options for a short-term replacement?*

- Every-type or spoon acrylic denture
- Immediate insertion adhesive/minimal preparation bridge
- In the very short term, the existing crown might be splinted to the adjacent teeth pending extraction.

■ *What are your options for the long-term replacement?*

Minimal preparation simple cantilever bridge replacing the lateral incisor with a retainer on the canine. This would require the carious lesion in the canine to be small and sufficient occlusal clearance for the retainer.

A conventional simple cantilever bridge using the canine as the abutment.

A conventional simple cantilever bridge using the upper left central incisor as the abutment. This would require a parallel-sided, cast or preformed post and core to support a single cantilever replacing the lateral incisor. Such a retainer is not ideal because using a post crowned tooth as a single abutment has a relatively high failure rate; indeed post retention is best avoided in all bridge designs. The failed root filling in the central incisor is also a problem. Retreatment would not produce a better root filling than the existing one which appears well condensed and as close to the apex as possible. Apicectomy will have to be considered for this tooth and if it is performed the root length available for a post will be reduced. Taken together with the time necessary to ensure apical healing, these factors exclude a replacement retained by the central incisor in the short term.

In the longer term this incisor might be usable as an abutment and if it were, the design could be further strengthened against rotation by using the mesial cavity in the canine for an inlay to act as a minor retainer for a fixed movable bridge.

A single tooth implant would be possible but a cautious approach is prudent in diabetes. This is not a complete contraindication to implants, but the possibility of delayed healing in diabetes, and the maxillary site (where implants have a reduced survival rate), mean that an implant might not be recommended. Further discussion of anterior single tooth implants will be found in Case 23.

CASE 12 Troublesome mouth ulcers

Summary

A 38-year-old woman with ulcers has noticed a recent exacerbation in their severity. You need to make a diagnosis and decide on suitable investigations and treatment.

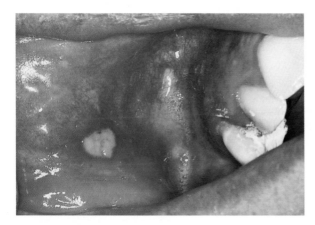

Fig. 12.1 The appearance of one ulcer.

HISTORY

Complaint

The patient complains of mouth ulcers which have been troubling her recently.

History of complaint

She has suffered occasional mouth ulcers, usually one at a time, over a period of more than 20 years. However, recently they seem to have become worse and she now has several. Normally she ignores them but, because she was attending your surgery for a filling, she thought she would ask whether anything could be done.

Medical history

The patient is otherwise fit and well.

■ *The patient has already provided several pieces of information of value for differential diagnosis. How do you assess her ulcers on the basis of the information available?*

The patient has noted an onset of ulceration early in life with recurrent attacks of single ulcers or small crops of ulcers. There are very many causes of oral ulceration but these appear to be **recurrent**, that is they appear periodically and heal completely between attacks. Recurrent ulceration has relatively few common causes.

■ *What are the common causes of recurrent oral ulceration?*

- Recurrent aphthous stomatitis (RAS)
  — Minor type
  — Herpetiform type
  — Major type
- Erythema multiforme
- Occasional cases of traumatic ulceration
- Ulcers associated with gastrointestinal disease.

■ *How will you differentiate between these conditions?*

Almost entirely on the basis of the findings in the history. Some features of the examination, blood tests or a biopsy may be helpful in certain cases, but the history is most important.

■ *What features of the ulceration would you ask about to determine the diagnosis? Explain why for each.*

See Table 12.1. This patient's answers are shown in the right-hand column.

■ *How are major and minor RAS differentiated?*

By severity rather than by any one feature alone. RAS may be labelled as major because of the size of the ulcers, their long duration or because they develop scarring on healing.

■ *From which type of ulcers does the patient appear to be suffering?*

She would appear to have typical minor RAS which has increased in severity recently.

EXAMINATION

Intraoral examination

■ *The appearance of one ulcer is shown in Figure 12.1. What do you see?*

There is an obvious ulcer on the anterior buccal mucosa. It is shallow, a few millimetres in diameter and has a slightly irregular but well-defined margin. The surrounding mucosa appears normal with only a narrow rim of erythema around the ulcer. There is a temporary restoration in the upper right first premolar and the ulcer would lie in approximately this region at rest.

Table 12.1 Features of ulceration

Feature	Reason	This patient's ulcers...
Site	Recurrent aphthous stomatitis (RAS) almost exclusively affects nonkeratinized mucosa. Erythema multiforme affects predominantly the vermilion border of lip, buccal mucosa and anterior mouth. Recurrent traumatic ulceration usually recurs at the same site.	... affect the labial mucosa and anterior buccal mucosa, especially in the sulci behind the lips. They never occur on the dorsal tongue or palate.
Size	Recurrent aphthous ulcer size depends on type. Minor ulcers are usually up to 8 mm in diameter, herpetiform 0.2 mm–3 mm, and major ulcers are larger than 1 cm, sometimes up to 3 or 4 cm in diameter.	... are usually 3–5 mm in diameter.
Duration of each ulcer	Minor RAS ulcers usually heal in approximately 10 days. Herpetiform ulcers may heal in about the same time or sometimes a shorter period (they are often smaller). Major RAS lesions may fail to heal for weeks or even months. Erythema multiforme is variable depending on severity and heals in 10–21 days.	... last a week or so before each ulcer heals.
Number of ulcers	Minor RAS lesions usually appear singly or in crops of 4–5 ulcers; major RAS lesions are fewer in number, often only one or two; herpetiform ulcers are numerous, from 30 to 100 at a time.	... are normally single, occasionally two to three develop at once. Recently there have been up to 5 at once.
Frequency of attacks	Frequency of attacks of RAS varies with severity. Ulcers may appear almost continuously or just once a year. Sometimes they coincide with menstruation. Erythema multiforme classically recurs at 6–8-week intervals in severe cases but the frequency may be only one or two attacks in a year.	... usually confined to one or two attacks a year but she has had three crops in the last 4 months.
Shape	RAS ulcers are usually round or oval and sharply defined, especially in the early stages. They may become more irregular as healing takes place. Ulcers in erythema multiforme are irregular and ragged and often poorly defined, merging with inflamed surrounding mucosa. Those on the lips are often covered by bloody fibrin sloughs.	... are round or oval.
Whether multiple ulcers develop synchronously or asynchronously	In RAS, ulcers may develop in crops within a few days of one another, or asynchronously. One crop may appear before another has healed. Herpetiform RAS lesions usually appear in crops together. In erythema multiforme allthe ulcers develop synchronously.	... usually appear within a few days of one another.
Are ulcers preceded by vesicles?	The presence of vesicles indicates possible viral infection or vesiculobullous disease. This fact may be helpful in the differential diagnosis of herpetiform ulcers which resemble viral ulcers but are not preceded by vesicles.	... have not been preceded by any vesicles, at least as far as the patient has been aware.
Age of onset	RAS usually has onset before or around adolescence. Erythema multiforme typically develops in the second or third decade.	... started with occasional ulcers in childhood and she has had occasional ulcers throughout her life.
Family history	Often present in RAS; not found in erythema multiforme.	... or ulcers like them do not appear to affect her parents. The patient's 7-year-old son occasionally has ulcers.
Exacerbating or relieving factors	None are usually detected for RAS, though an ulcer may develop at a site of minor trauma, complicating the differential diagnosis if the ulcers are very infrequent. Stress often appears to precipitate attacks of RAS. Erythema multiforme may be triggered by a drug, viral or other infection, classically 10 days before the ulcers appear. Often no trigger is identified.	... occasionally develop where she bites herself or knocks her mucosa with a toothbrush.

When you examine the patient you find two more ulcers. One is 2 mm in diameter and lies in the lower labial sulcus on the alveolar mucosa adjacent to the lower right canine. A third ulcer, also 3 mm in diameter, lies on the upper left buccal mucosa anterior to the parotid papilla. They appear to be identical to the ulcer shown.

■ *What can you deduce from these appearances?*

The appearances are not particularly helpful in differential diagnosis but are typical of those seen in minor recurrent aphthous stomatitis. The slightly irregular outline of the largest ulcer indicates early healing. The ulcers are not at all suggestive of erythema multiforme.

If you were able to examine the mouth you would find that there is no evidence of scarring in the common ulcer sites, which would have suggested the major form of RAS. The mucosa is otherwise healthy excluding the possibility of chronic ulceration in a mucosal disease, such as lichen planus or a vesiculobullous disease. The normal mucosa at sites of previous ulcers confirms that the ulceration is indeed recurrent.

DIAGNOSIS

■ *What is your diagnosis and what would you do next?*

The diagnosis is recurrent aphthous stomatitis of the minor form. The next step is to exclude the possibility that the ulcers are associated with an underlying condition.

■ *With what underlying conditions/causes may RAS be associated?*

- Iron deficiency
- Vitamin deficiency, particularly B_{12} and folate
- Gastrointestinal disease
- Behçet's disease
- Smoking cessation.

■ *What features of the ulcers themselves might indicate the presence of an underlying predisposing condition?*

Any feature in the history or examination which is atypical for the type of RAS should raise suspicion of an underlying condition. In particular, the following should trigger a search for underlying predisposing causes:
- Onset after the second decade
- Increase in ulcer size, duration, symptoms or severity
- Marked periulcer erythema.

■ *How would you investigate the possibility of an underlying condition?*

Iron deficiency is relatively common. Check for known history of anaemia. Question the patient about common causes of iron-deficiency anaemia, including menorrhagia and gastrointestinal bleeding (peptic ulcer, hiatus hernia, inflammatory bowel disease and haemorrhoids). Check that a balanced and varied diet is consumed, even though dietary deficiency is rare. Perform blood tests or refer the patient to her medical practitioner to check for microcytosis and to determine haemoglobin and red cell/haemoglobin indices. Ulcers may be associated with minor degrees of iron deficiency which are insufficient to cause anaemia and sensitive tests for iron depletion are required. Serum ferritin, which reflects body iron stores, is the ideal test.

Vitamin deficiencies associated with aphthous stomatitis are usually of folate or B_{12}. Check that a balanced and varied diet is consumed and that there is no gastrointestinal disease to reduce absorption of folate. Exclude dietary deficiency of B_{12} by asking about pernicious anaemia and gastrointestinal disease and confirming that the diet is adequate, particularly if a strict vegetarian diet is consumed. Perform blood tests for mean cell volume (increased in deficiency) and assay serum or erythrocyte folate level and serum B_{12}.

Gastrointestinal disease exacerbates RAS because of reduced absorption of iron, folate and B_{12}. Ask about both diarrhoea and constipation, abdominal cramps, weight loss and blood in stools and check the medical history.

Gastrointestinal diseases are also associated with other types of oral ulceration. Sometimes these ulcers are recurrent but their appearances are usually characteristic and they are most unlikely to be mistaken for ulcers of RAS. Large leathery ulcers, multiple pustules and irregular haemorrhagic ulcers are very occasionally seen in ulcerative colitis, linear ulcers with hyperplastic margins in Crohn's disease and herpetiform-type ulcers in coeliac disease.

Behçet's disease is rare but can occasionally present with oral ulcers. Patients may suffer from a broad spectrum of signs and symptoms and should be questioned about genital ulcers on mucosa or skin, rashes including erythema nodosum or pustules, arthritis of large joints, venous thrombosis and bowel symptoms. Ocular signs including uveitis and conjunctivitis are found in a minority of patients and these, and central nervous system symptoms, are serious. There are no specific tests for Behçet's disease (though HLA typing may help identify those at risk from ocular disease). A biopsy of an oral ulcer may be helpful because it can demonstrate the underlying vasculitis which accounts for many of the manifestations.

Smoking cessation is excluded by questioning. It sometimes exacerbates ulceration but starting smoking again does not usually induce remission.

TREATMENT

■ *What treatments are available and which would you suggest?*

Many treatments are available. Unfortunately none is highly effective in all patients and treatment must be selected to suit individual cases. Reassurance is an important part of treatment in minor RAS. Tell the patient that RAS is very common, but is a 'nuisance' condition rather than serious or infectious and warn her that:

- no one treatment is consistently effective;
- she may need to try several treatments before she finds one which works well for her;
- treatments are not completely effective, and they should only be expected to moderate the symptoms and sometimes the frequency of ulcers;
- the aim of treatment should be to make the ulcers bearable.

If an underlying condition such as iron deficiency is detected, its correction will probably reduce their severity but will not cure the ulcers completely.

Treatments available are shown in Table 12.2.

For this patient, the most important factor is to exclude underlying causes and iron deficiency is the most likely. Treatment of underlying deficiency may reduce the ulcer severity so that the patient can again ignore her ulcers. In the meantime a mouthwash or hydrocortisone pellets would appear to be suitable as a first-line treatment though the patient might also be encouraged to try some of the many nonprescription preparations available.

Table 12.2 Treatments for minor RAS

Treatment	Indications
No treatment	Probably the best option for occasional ulcers.
Covering agents, e.g. Orabase	Good for infrequent ulcers anteriorly in the buccal and labial mucosa, ideally single ulcers. Use is difficult and the patient must be capable of some dexterity.
Anti-inflammatory/analgesic mouthwash, e.g. benzydamine Antiseptic mouthwashes, e.g. chlorhexidine.	Both types of mouthwash are useful when ulcers affect a range of oral sites not accessible to covering pastes. In general not highly effective but may reduce pain directly or by reducing infection of the ulcer surface. Popular with most patients.
Low potency topical steroid pellets such as hydrocortisone (Corlan) and steroid in Orabase such as triamcinolone (Adcortyl in Orabase)	Ulcers must be at sites where the pellet can be left to dissolve or Orabase applied, usually in the sulci. Useful first-line treatment if the ulcer-free period is longer than 1 month and may reduce frequency in some patients.
Steroid mouthwashes, e.g. betamethasone	Used when ulcers affect a range of sites and are of sufficient severity to merit a therapeutic treatment. Potent, not available to general dental practitioners in the UK. Patient must dissolve tablets to make fresh mouthwash.
Steroid aerosols, e.g. budesonide	Useful when a more potent steroid must be delivered to a single site. Potent, not available to general dental practitioners in the UK.
Systemic drugs, steroids, colchicine	For severe cases and Behçet's disease refractory to other treatments. Potent, not available to general dental practitioners in the UK.

In addition, simple advice may help make ulcers bearable: avoid spicy foods, acidic fruit juices and carbonated drinks; consider drinking with a straw when ulcers are present; avoid sharp foods such as crisps, and astringent toothpastes or those with irritant flavourings or detergents.

■ *The patient asks whether the lip ulcer could be caused by the temporary restoration in the adjacent tooth. What is your opinion?*

No. This is most unlikely. The history of RAS is so typical that the diagnosis is not in doubt. Reactions to dental materials are not associated with ulcers of this type. However, recurrent aphthous ulcers often develop at the sites of minor trauma. Trauma either during restoration, from a sharp edge or from biting while the mucosa was anaesthetized might well explain the location of this particular ulcer.

13 A lump in the neck

Summary

A 55-year-old man presents to your oral and maxillofacial surgery department clinic with a lump on the left side of the neck. You must make a diagnosis.

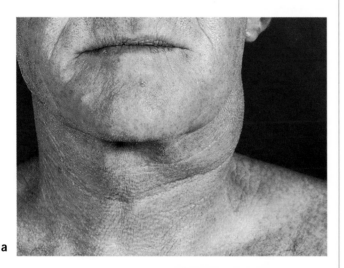

a

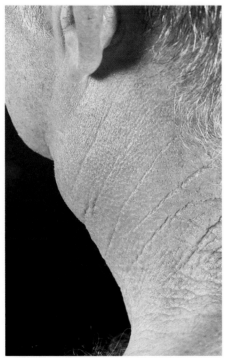

b

Fig. 13.1 a and **b** The appearance of the swelling.

Complaint

The patient complains of the lump and notices some discomfort on swallowing, as if something is stuck in his throat. He assumes the lump is the cause.

History of present complaint

He thinks he first noticed the lump about 3 months ago. It has always been painless and is slowly enlarging. The discomfort on swallowing is of recent onset.

Medical history

The patient is otherwise fit and well. He smokes 20 cigarettes per day and drinks 10 units of alcohol each week as beer.

Extraoral examination

The appearance of the swelling is shown in Figure 13.1.

■ *What do you see? What is the likely origin of the mass?*

There is a swelling just anterior to the anterior border of the sternomastoid muscle and below and behind the angle of the mandible. It is several centimetres in diameter and extends forwards below the angle of the mandible towards the submandibular region. The overlying skin does not appear to be inflamed.

The lesion lies over the deep cervical lymph node chain and could well arise from a cervical lymph node. It is too low and too far posterior to be arising from the submandibular gland and probably too low to have arisen in the lower pole of the parotid gland. Other soft tissues of the neck could be the origin, but a lymph node is the most likely cause.

If you could palpate the lesion you would find that it is approximately 8 cm by 6 cm in size and feels firm on palpation, possibly slightly fluctuant. It is mobile, not fixed to the overlying skin or deep structures. The patient does not notice any tenderness on palpation. There are no other swellings or enlarged lymph nodes palpable on either side of the neck.

Intraoral examination

The submandibular glands are palpable bimanually and appear symmetrical. Both are mobile and clearly separate from the swelling which lies posterior to the gland.

The patient's mouth has been well restored in the past but suffers from recent neglect and several carious cavities are visible. There is no significant periodontal disease with most probing depths less than 5 mm and no mobile teeth. The lower left first permanent molar has lost a large restoration and has extensive caries. There is no soft tissue swelling, sinus or tenderness in the sulcus adjacent to the apices of the roots. The tooth is not tender to percussion. The oral mucosa appears normal, and the tonsils appear to be symmetrical.

DIFFERENTIAL DIAGNOSIS

■ *What are the most likely causes of this lump and why?*

Metastatic malignancy appears likely and this lesion is so typical of a cervical lymph node metastasis that it must be considered to be malignant until proved otherwise. The combination of features suggestive of metastasis is the patient's age (should be considered a possible cause in any patient aged over 45), the site (consistent with a cervical lymph node), the firm consistency and lack of tenderness. Fixation to the skin or other structures would be almost conclusive of malignancy but is a late sign. The patient is a smoker and drinker and so has an increased risk of malignancy. Either a squamous carcinoma or adenocarcinoma are likely. Melanoma and other malignancies are further possible causes.

Lymphadenitis secondary to a local cause is common and so must be considered. However there is no tenderness on palpation to suggest an inflammatory cause. If this were a reactive inflammatory enlargement, the most likely source of

infection would be a dental, pharyngeal or skin infection. The patient has a potential source of dental infection in the lower left first permanent molar but the tooth is not tender to percussion nor associated with overt infection, making it an unlikely cause.

Tuberculosis needs to be considered both as a possible diagnosis and as a factor affecting management. Most patients with cervical lymph node enlargement caused by tuberculosis have reactivation ('secondary' or post-primary) tuberculosis in which a previous quiescent infection becomes reactivated. This localized infection may or may not be accompanied by pulmonary disease though there may be radiological evidence of past tuberculosis on chest radiograph. Cervical tuberculous lymphadenitis is common in those from the Indian subcontinent. Atypical mycobacterial infection is a disease which often affects the cervical lymph nodes but is almost always seen in children or the immunosuppressed.

■ *Which additional but less likely causes need to be considered whenever a patient complains of an enlargement at this site? Why are they unlikely causes in this case?*

Numerous lesions could arise at this site and it is not useful to list them all. A number of possible causes (Table 13.1) merit consideration, either because they are common, easily excluded or cause significant morbidity.

Table 13.1 Further possible causes of the enlargement

Cause		Reasons
Developmental causes	Branchial cyst	Branchial cysts develop at this site. They usually present in childhood or early adulthood but can on occasion be asymptomatic for many years and present late with infection. However, 55 years of age would be extremely late and a metastatic malignancy is a much more likely cause. Cystic change in metastatic carcinoma in lymph nodes is a well recognized finding and fluctuance can be misinterpreted as indicating a benign cyst such as a branchial cyst.
Infectious causes	Cat scratch disease, toxoplasmosis, brucellosis, glandular fever	These are less common causes of cervical lymphadenopathy in this age group. All usually cause enlargement of several nodes, often bilaterally. Toxoplasmosis and glandular fever usually affect young adults. Cat scratch disease may present with a single markedly enlarged node. Exposure to cats or other pets or history of a primary skin infection at the site of a scratch aids diagnosis. Serological tests allow the diagnosis of cat scratch disease, toxoplasmosis and brucellosis. Of these conditions, only cat scratch disease is a conceivable cause for this swelling and the likelihood is low.
	HIV infection	Should always be considered in chronic lymph node enlargement but causes generalized lymphadenopathy. May be accompanied by signs of immunosuppression. A most unlikely diagnosis for this presentation.
Inflammatory causes	Sarcoidosis	Another cause of generalized lymphadenopathy or enlargement of a group of nodes. More common in the 20–40 age group. African–Americans, West Indian and Irish immigrants to the UK are at particular risk. Usually accompanied by other signs which aid diagnosis. An unlikely cause for this patient's swelling.
Benign neoplasms	Salivary gland neoplasm	The tail of the parotid gland extends low into the neck, to just below and behind the angle of the mandible. This lesion does not appear to be in the correct site for a parotid gland origin but the possibility of a benign salivary neoplasm might be considered. A Warthin's tumour or pleomorphic adenoma would be the most likely possibilities because they are commonest.
	Carotid body tumour (paraganglioma)	These arise from the carotid body at the carotid bifurcation and cause a swelling just in front of the sternomastoid muscle but slightly higher than the present swelling. They are rare, affect the 30–60-year-old age group and are sometimes bilateral. Though an unusual cervical swelling, the accompanying pulsation, thrill or bruit from the carotid blood supply aids diagnosis. The lesion is mobile horizontally but not vertically because it is attached to the carotid artery. An unlikely cause for this patient's swelling.
	Other benign soft tissue neoplasm	Many are possible, arising from muscle, nerve, fat or fibrous tissue. None merits singling out as a possible cause in this case.
Other primary malignant neoplasms	Lymphoma	An enlarged lymph node in the deep cervical lymph chain could be the first presentation of lymphoma. Non-Hodgkin's lymphoma would be the most likely type in a patient of this age. However, enlarged lymph nodes in lymphoma are almost always multiple and feel rubbery. The presence of such a large discrete lesion without other enlarged lymph nodes almost completely excludes lymphoma.

Table 13.2 Techniques for obtaining tissue

Investigation	Advantages	Disadvantages
Fine-needle aspiration biopsy/cytology (FNA or FNAB)	The least invasive procedure which can provide a sample of the lesional tissue. FNA does not risk seeding tumour or tuberculosis into the tissues of the neck. Rapid Readily repeated if fails. Leaves no scar	It is possible to miss the lesion when inserting the needle. If this is likely to be a problem, the procedure can be performed under ultrasound or radiological guidance. Provides only a small sample and definitive diagnosis on cytology may not be possible (though a sufficiently accurate diagnosis to plan treatment may be provided).
Incisional biopsy	Readily performed and provides a large tissue sample which will almost certainly be sufficient for diagnosis. In lymphoma, a lymph node is usually required for classification of disease. (However, the neck is not the favoured site for reasons of appearance and another node would probably be sampled.)	If the lesion were malignant it would probably be spread into the tissues of the neck, making subsequent surgical treatment very difficult, if not impossible. This complication can be minimized by taking the biopsy from an area which would later be excised. However, spread into the tissue planes of the neck cannot be reliably prevented. Risk to adjacent structures in the neck

Table 13.3 Other investigations

Investigation	Reason
Vitality tests	To search for dental causes of infection
Radiographs of teeth on left side	To search for a dental infectious cause and provide information to plan necessary dental treatment.
Sialogram	To determine whether the mass is within the submandibular or parotid glands.
Chest radiograph	To search for metastasis in lungs, or for evidence of tuberculosis.
Serology	Viral titres and specific tests to determine potential infectious causes such as cat scratch fever.
Ultrasound scan	To determine the lesion's relationship to the salivary glands; determine its extent, and whether it is cystic; to find out whether other masses or enlarged lymph nodes are present.
CT/MRI scan/PET scan	To localize the lesion and its relationships to normal tissues. Unnecessary at this stage. May be required later to plan treatment when diagnosis is established.

INVESTIGATIONS

■ *What is the most important investigation? Which methods might be used and what are their advantages and disadvantages?*

The critical requirement when malignancy is suspected is to obtain tissue speedily for microscopic diagnosis. All other investigations are less important at this stage. Two techniques are in common use, the fine-needle aspiration biopsy and the surgical incisional biopsy (Table 13.2).

■ *What other investigations might be performed, either now or at a later date? Why?*

See Table 13.3.

In this case a suitable combination of investigations would be fine-needle aspiration, dental radiographs, vitality tests and possibly ultrasound scan. The sialogram would have been performed if a salivary origin had been thought possible after clinical examination.

The lower first molar was nonvital and a periapical radiograph revealed apical radiolucency. The smear from a fine-needle aspirate is shown in Figure 13.2.

■ *What does the fine-needle aspirate show and how do you interpret the appearances?*

The aspirate shows cells from the lesion spread as a single layer and stained with the Papanicolaou stain. This stains

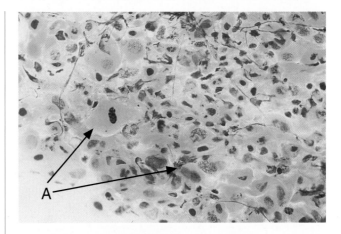

Fig. 13.2 Fine-needle aspirate from the lesion.

nuclei dark blue, keratin orange and the cytoplasm of nonkeratinized epithelial cells turquoise. The cells are almost all epithelial as shown by their prominent cytoplasm and by the presence of keratinization (arrowed A) in some of them. The larger cells have angulate polygonal cytoplasm typical of squamous epithelial cells. The nuclei of the cells range markedly in size from small hyperchromatic nuclei to very large irregular nuclei. At higher power the chromatin pattern is coarse. These features indicate malignancy and the keratinized cells indicate that this is a squamous carcinoma. Many normal lymphocytes were found elsewhere on the slide. This indicates that the carcinoma is in a lymph node and is therefore a metastasis.

DIAGNOSIS

The patient has metastatic squamous carcinoma, almost certainly in a cervical lymph node.

■ *What are the possible sites for the primary malignant neoplasm?*

Any site in the drainage area of the lymph node in which squamous carcinoma may develop.

Oral mucosa, particularly ventrolateral tongue, floor of mouth, soft palate, fauces or retromolar mucosa

Pharynx, nasopharynx or oropharynx

Tonsil

Maxillary sinus

Facial skin and scalp

Salivary glands

■ *What would you do to localize the primary carcinoma?*

- Check history for previous known malignant disease.
- Re-examine for symptoms or signs of possible primary carcinomas.
- Upper aerodigestive tract endoscopy under general anaesthesia.

In this case, endoscopy revealed an ulcerated mass in the pharynx near the base of the tongue, and biopsy revealed squamous cell carcinoma.

■ *What would you do if a primary carcinoma is not identified?*

During endoscopy, blind biopsy of the nasopharynx and ipsilateral tonsillectomy may reveal an unsuspected small carcinoma. If this fails to identify the primary then the search will have to be widened, intially to other common sites for squamous carcinoma, such as lung, and then to the whole body. Very occasionally no primary lesion is found.

TREATMENT

■ *What are the treatment options assuming a primary is identified in the head and neck?*

The treatment of choice for primary head and neck squamous carcinoma with lymph node involvement is surgical resection, with subsequent radiotherapy in selected cases to eradicate any possible residual disease. Radiotherapy is always given if the carcinoma is found to have spread outside the capsule of lymph nodes in which metastases have seeded (extracapsular spread). Radiotherapy alone would be used in selected cases such as small tongue carcinomas, for palliation in advanced carcinoma or when patients refuse surgery. Surgery would usually involve the en bloc removal of the primary site and lymph nodes from the deep cervical chain in continuity (block dissection of neck). Reconstruction using local, distant or free flaps may be required.

Chemotherapy and immunotherapy are of little benefit in squamous carcinoma of the head and neck.

ANOTHER POSSIBILITY

■ *If the fine-needle aspirate had shown adenocarcinoma or poorly differentiated carcinoma, which possible primary sites would have required investigation?*

Adenocarcinoma (carcinoma showing glandular differentiation) might well have arisen in the breast, lung or prostate. The thyroid, salivary glands and minor mucous glands in the upper aerodigestive tract would also be possible primary sites. A poorly differentiated carcinoma could have metastasized from any of the squamous carcinoma or adenocarcinoma primary sites.

The stomach is a further possible source and a low cervical metastasis on the left side is a recognized presentation. However, in this case the swelling is too high in the neck to have arisen from the stomach.

■ *Why does a gastrointestinal carcinoma sometimes metastasize to the left side of the neck?*

Lymph from the oesophagus and the upper part of the stomach drains upwards in the thoracic duct which enters the lower end of the internal jugular vein. There is a rather variable anatomy at the site and often the subclavian and internal jugular lymph trunks join the thoracic duct rather than the internal jugular vein. In this situation, malignant cells draining up the thoracic duct can be carried a short distance into the lymphatics of the neck by retrograde flow (because the lymphatics are at a low and fluctuating pressure). Such cells can seed metastases in the lymph nodes just above the clavicle (Virchow's node).

CASE 14

Trauma to an immature incisor

Summary

An 8-year-old girl has fractured her upper right permanent central incisor tooth.

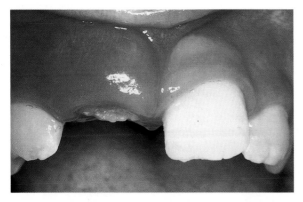

Fig. 14.1 The patient's anterior dentition on presentation.

HISTORY

Complaint

The child is brought in as an emergency by her mother, complaining of a broken front tooth.

History of complaint

Two hours prior to presentation the child had slipped at school, hitting her mouth. One front tooth appears to be broken.

Medical history

The child suffers mild asthma, but is otherwise healthy.

Dental history

The child has attended the dentist irregularly but has had no caries and has no experience of operative dentistry. Her mother states that the broken tooth had not appeared normal and may have been decayed.

■ *What additional questions would you ask and why?*

Did the patient lose consciousness? This would indicate a relatively severe blow to the head and might indicate significant intracranial trauma. If the patient lost consciousness, even for a short period, they should be referred to hospital where they would almost certainly be admitted for 24 hours of observation. In this case the patient did not lose consciousness.

Was a piece of the tooth broken off and was it found? Missing fragments of teeth may have been inhaled, swallowed, embedded in the lip or lost. If a fragment has been found it must be matched to the fracture to determine whether other pieces remain missing and the patient investigated to locate and remove the pieces. In this case no fragment was found.

Has the patient suffered trauma previously? Previous trauma to this tooth could have resulted in arrested root development, disturbed crown formation or pathological mobility prior to this incident, depending on the age and stage of dental development at the time. Such changes could affect treatment and might explain the parent's observation that the tooth was not normal. In this case no previous trauma could be recalled by the parent.

Was the damaged tooth fully erupted before the accident? In early mixed dentition, incisors on opposite sides of the mouth may be at different stages of eruption. At this age it would be expected that eruption would be complete but there is wide variation in eruption date and rate. It would be possible to misinterpret incomplete eruption as an intrusion injury if the original degree of eruption were not known. In this case, the child's mother reported that both front teeth were fully erupted.

What object or surface did the child hit with her mouth? Injury on surfaces such as playgrounds, roads and pavements carries the risk of contaminating the wound with dirty particulate material. Sometimes such foreign material even enters intraoral wounds. Thorough debridement would then be required. It would also be necessary to check the child's immunization status for tetanus prophylaxis and arrange a booster dose if required. In this case, the child hit the edge of a table.

EXAMINATION

Extraoral examination

The child is distressed but is readily examined. There is some slight swelling of the upper lip but no external abrasions or lacerations.

Intraoral examination

■ *The appearances of the teeth are shown in Figure 14.1. What do you see?*

The gingival tissues labial to the upper right permanent central incisor are erythematous and swollen. The crown of the tooth appears missing and less than 1 mm of the tooth is visible above the level of the gingiva. The visible fragment appears to be an intact incisal edge rather than a fractured enamel or root surface. The other upper incisors show mild hypoplasia of the labial enamel in the incisal third of the crown.

If you were able to examine the patient you would find that the palatal gingiva of the upper right central incisor are also red and swollen. The remainder of the dentition is caries-free. There are no lacerations in the mucosa of the inner aspect of the lip.

■ *What additional examinations(s) would you perform?*

Injury to the adjacent incisors and teeth in the lower labial segment should be investigated. Vitality, mobility, tenderness to percussion and fractures should be noted. A periodontal probe should be gently inserted into the labial gingival sulcus to confirm or exclude the presence of a deep pseudo-pocket which would indicate traumatic displacement.

■ *Having completed the examination, what question should the examining dentist keep in the back of their mind? Explain why.*

Are the injuries seen consistent with the history given? If not, inconsistencies in the history should be probed by further gentle questioning. While children are often reluctant to offer an accurate account of minor accidents, significant inconsistencies or evasive responses by the parent or child should raise suspicion of nonaccidental injury. Such suspicions should be discussed with a colleague if possible and, if felt to be justified, with the patient's general medical practitioner or the local Child Protection Advisor.

■ *What features in the history and examination would lead to suspicion of nonaccidental injury?*

History of repeated trauma (dental and facial injury, but also limb fractures)

Presenting injury not consistent with history given

Child's account varies significantly from parental account

History changed over course of initial consultation or review visits, evasive answers to questions

Delayed presentation

Bruises, abrasions or other soft tissue lesions apparently sustained over a period of time (for instance at different stages of healing) which are not accounted for by the presenting injury

DIFFERENTIAL DIAGNOSIS

■ *What is your initial differential diagnosis?*

There are two main possibilities, either the central incisor has been almost completely intruded (intrusive luxation) or its crown has been fractured horizontally at gingival level. The appearance in the figure indicates that this is almost certainly an intrusion luxation because the visible tooth is an intact incisal edge rather than a fractured root.

INVESTIGATIONS

■ *What investigations would you perform? Explain why for each.*

Radiographs are required to visualize the intruded/fractured tooth and to assess damage to it and the adjacent teeth. Periapical views should be taken of all upper incisors to detect possible root fracture and to assess the stage of root development of the incisors. In intrusion injuries the force of the blow is directed upwards so that it is unlikely that the lower incisors have been damaged. However, if the upper incisor turns out to be fractured then the lower incisors should also be radiographed to exclude root fracture. The periapical view of the upper right central incisor is shown in Figure 14.2.

Tests of vitality of all incisors are required. If the patient is sufficiently composed to allow it, all the incisors should be checked for vitality, preferably by electric pulp testing. Teeth recently subjected to trauma may not respond to testing ('concussion') and testing teeth with open apices may give an artificially low reading. However, it is important to take a baseline reading soon after the injury so that if vitality does not recover, treatment may be instituted without delay.

■ *The periapical radiograph is shown in Figure 14.2. What does the radiograph show?*

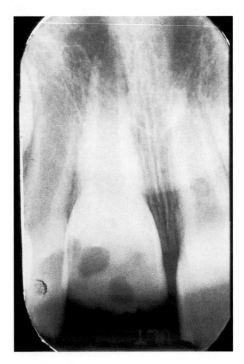

Fig. 14.2 Periapical radiograph.

The radiograph shows a severe intrusive luxation of the maxillary right permanent incisor. The periodontal ligament space is indistinct or obliterated in parts. There is no crown or root fracture visible, and the root is immature with a wide open apex. A peculiar feature on the film is the small circular radiolucent areas on the crown of the intruded tooth. These are well demarcated and smooth in outline.

■ *What could these radiolucent areas be?*

The lesions are relatively radiolucent and lie towards the incisal edge where enamel rather than dentine is responsible for the radiopacity of the tooth. This suggests that missing enamel is likely to be the cause. The patient's mother mentioned that the tooth had always appeared decayed and causes predating the current injury are the most likely. A number might be considered:

Cause	Merits as a diagnosis
Loss of enamel/ dentine as a direct result of the trauma	Such an injury would be unusual and the circular pattern is difficult to explain.
Dental caries	Caries in this distribution also seems unlikely. Labial surface caries is usually found following the gingival margin in individuals with poor oral hygiene. This child is caries-free and has good oral hygiene.
Enamel hypoplasia	Could affect single or multiple teeth. Hypoplasia was noted in the incisal third of the enamel of the adjacent teeth. Hypoplasia could not result from the present injury because the teeth were erupted.
Resorption defects	These are a possibility but the distribution would be unusual and some cause, such as previous injury, might be expected. Resorption could not occur so rapidly after the current intrusion but may be seen on the root surface some months following an intrusive luxation.

Enamel hypoplasia would appear to be the most likely cause.

■ *Why is there a horizontal dark line on the radiograph across the crown of the upper left central and upper right lateral incisor?*

It is the edge of the soft tissue shadow of the upper lip.

DIAGNOSIS

■ *What is your final diagnosis?*

The patient has an intrusive luxation to the permanent central incisor. This tooth also has several discrete hypoplastic enamel defects which were present before the accident.

TREATMENT

■ *What types of tissue injury result from intrusion and what are their complications?*

Injury	Complication
Crushing and rupture of the periodontal fibres	Bacterial infection or inflammation tracking along the periodontal ligament. Increased risk of root resorption. Weakened periodontal attachment.

Injury	Complication
Crushing, devitalization and scraping off of cementum	Transient surface root resorption with the possibility of more extensive external resorption and ankylosis in the longer term.
Crushing of the apical neurovascular bundle (and the pulp itself in immature teeth)	Loss of pulp vitality.

■ *Will the tooth re-erupt or should it be surgically repositioned?*

All mature teeth (closed apex) and over 60% of immature teeth become nonvital as a result of intrusive luxation. Therefore, it is advisable to reposition the tooth as rapidly as possible so that access to the pulp chamber can be facilitated before pulp necrosis occurs. Intruded teeth with open apices do have the potential for re-eruption, but if this has not commenced within 1 week, intervention is required. There is at present no evidence to indicate the optimal treatment for the intrusive luxation of permanent teeth. Given sufficient cooperation, immediate surgical repositioning of the tooth will immediately restore the appearance. This should be followed by a short period of splinting of 7–10 days. This option may, however, increase the likelihood of external root resorption and loss of marginal bone support. Relatively rapid orthodontic extrusion over a period of 3–4 weeks is considered less traumatic and less likely to induce resorption.

■ *What immediate treatment is indicated?*

Immediate treatment aims to prevent subsequent external root resorption, preserve marginal bone support and prevent sepsis. Teeth with a closed apex should be treated by immediate pulp extirpation and placement of a non-setting calcium hydroxide root canal dressing. Immature teeth should be monitored for spontaneous re-eruption and loss of vitality. A 5-day course of systemic antibiotics should be prescribed, and the false gingival pocket surrounding the intruded crown gently irrigated with chlorhexidine.

■ *What follow up should you arrange?*

Follow-up period	Reason
1 week	To monitor spontaneous eruption and vitality of immature teeth, or to remove the splint and change the calcium hydroxide paste in a tooth treated by immediate repositioning.
3 weeks and 6 months	To continue monitoring spontaneous re-eruption of an immature tooth. Replace calcium hydroxide dressing. Radiograph.
6-monthly and then annually for several years	To observe for delayed onset of external root resorption.

In this case, spontaneous eruption was awaited, but was very slow. Electric pulp testing indicated early pulp necrosis. The tooth was then extruded rapidly with a simple orthodontic appliance engaged on to a bracket attached to the labial surface of the intruded tooth. As soon as there was adequate access to the pulp chamber, the necrotic pulp was extirpated, the canal cleaned and obturated with non-setting calcium hydroxide paste. The appearance of the extruded tooth is shown in Figure 14.3 and it confirms the diagnosis of enamel hypoplasia made radiographically.

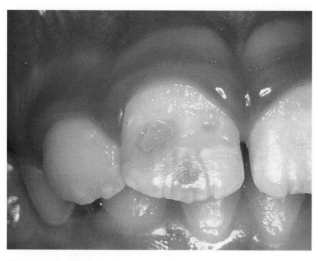

Fig. 14.3 Appearance of the extruded upper right central incisor.

■ *How would your management have differed if the patient had been a 3-year-old child with an intruded deciduous incisor?*

Mild intrusive luxation injuries in the deciduous dentition may be treated with reassurance and observation though parents should always be warned that damage to the permanent successor is common. Partial or sometimes total re-eruption over the following months is usual.

However, extraction should be performed without delay if a combination of periapical and lateral radiographs demonstrate that the deciduous tooth has impinged on the follicle of the underlying tooth or if there is subsequent loss of vitality. As in the permanent dentition, vitality must be monitored carefully if the apex is closed at the time of injury. Pulp tests in young children are often unreliable because of lack of understanding, and a close watch must be kept for colour change.

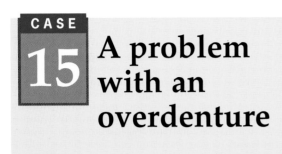

A problem with an overdenture

Summary

A 67-year-old lady is referred to your general dental practice complaining that her denture has never 'seemed right' from the day it was fitted.

HISTORY

Complaint

The patient complains that a small filling has recently been lost from one of the upper canine roots below her overdenture. However, it quickly becomes clear that this has caused no symptoms (the tooth is root-treated) and that she is dissatisfied primarily with her upper complete overdenture. She can wear the denture in the morning, but by about three o'clock in the afternoon it becomes too uncomfortable and if she is at home she likes to take it out.

History of complaint

The patient successfully wore an acrylic upper partial denture until 6 months ago, but failure of restorations and root treatments led to loss of several upper teeth. She was provided with an upper overdenture on the two retained upper canine roots. The denture was fitted 3 months ago, reviewed on four occasions and minor adjustments were made to the base extension. The patient is happy with the retention and fit of the denture. It does not move during eating. She reports no problem with her lower teeth.

Medical history

The patient is taking half an aspirin a day following a myocardial infarction.

EXAMINATION

Extraoral examination

There is no lymphadenopathy. The temporomandibular joint is free of crepitus and clicks, and no muscle tenderness can be elicited in the muscles of mastication. With the denture in place, there is no facial asymmetry. The patient has a slightly open lip posture at rest.

Intraoral examination

The patient has a well-developed upper alveolar ridge with limited resorption consistent with the relatively recent loss of several upper teeth. There is slight redness of the palate under the denture-bearing area, but the ridge is not tender on palpation at any site and there is no bleeding on probing around the canine roots and no detectable sinus. One of the root-treated canine teeth has lost a small restoration from the access cavity. The remainder of the oral mucosa is normal.

There is an almost complete lower arch of natural teeth. These are adequately restored, many with large amalgam restorations, and there is no caries. The occlusal plane is relatively even. There has been slight mesial tipping of the lower second molars as a result of loss of both first molars.

The denture appears clean and without obvious defects and there is a definite post dam along its posterior margin.

■ *On the basis of what you know so far, what are the likely diagnoses and why?*

The patient has successfully worn a denture and the transition to an overdenture from an upper acrylic partial denture should have been relatively straightforward. It might have been more difficult if the previous denture had been metal-based. If the patient has persevered for 3 months without success she almost certainly has a valid complaint.

There appears to be no problem of displacement of the denture during eating, speaking or other facial movements. This makes it unlikely that the overdenture is poorly adapted, overextended or that the teeth lie outside the neutral zone. Occlusal discrepancies of some kind would appear to be the most likely cause and the vagueness of the complaint, predominantly inability to tolerate the denture, is consistent with an occlusal problem. A further reason to suspect an occlusal problem is the difficulty arising from a complete upper denture occluding against a lower natural arch.

It must also be borne in mind that some denture patients are particularly conscious of appearance and the construction of dentures which satisfy the expectations of such patients can be very demanding. Sometimes a mismatch between the denture appearance and desired facial self-image may manifest as dislike of the denture or complaints about relatively minor features. There is always a potential cosmetic problem of an overcontoured labial flange when canine roots support an upper overdenture because the roots preserve the labial face of the alveolar bone.

■ *What specific features of the dentures would you examine and how?*

All features of the denture should be reviewed (Table 15.1). Denture complaints may be multifactorial and only by examining all features can an accurate diagnosis be made.

Having examined the patient you find that the denture is correctly extended, stable and retentive. The denture was not displaced on lateral excursion. This leaves the vertical dimension as the most likely cause of an occlusal problem.

Table 15.1 Examination of the denture

Feature	Method
Check base extension. Is the denture correctly extended into the sulcus?	This is done visually where possible, checking the relationship between the denture border, sulcus depth and soft tissue mobility at rest and under tension. In less visible areas, such as lateral to the tuberosity, palpation may be required.
Does the posterior border extend back to the vibrating area?	Identify the vibrating area by observing the soft tissue moving when the patient says 'Ahhh' and/or apply pressure with a blunt instrument such as a ball-ended burnisher to define the extent of displaceable tissue.
Is the denture retentive?	Check by pulling down on the upper denture in the premolar region. Check retention of the post dam by trying to displace the denture with forward pressure behind the anterior teeth.
Is there close adaptation of the denture base to the mucosa?	Look at the fit surface and check for voids between tissue and denture with a disclosing material such as a low viscosity silicone.
Make an assessment of the occlusal vertical dimension and patient's rest vertical dimension	Measure the facial height at rest and with the denture in occlusion. Subtract to identify the freeway space. (See below.)
Is the occlusion correct in retruded position?	Check whether the denture meets the natural teeth correctly in retruded position. Are there any premature contacts?
Are the natural teeth affecting the occlusal plane significantly?	Check the occlusal plane to ensure that the natural standing teeth do not place excessive destabilizing forces on the prosthesis. Assess in particular whether the denture is stable on lateral excursive movements.
Appearance	Check tooth shade, shape and set up. Carefully question the patient as to whether they are satisfied with the appearance. Check the soft tissue support provided by the denture, particularly over the canine roots.
*If there were a **lower** complete denture, you should check to ensure that the teeth lie in the neutral zone, and for denture stability. (Not directly relevant in this case.)*	*Look at the denture when the patient's mouth is half-open. Is the lower denture displaced by the tongue or lips?*

■ *What methods can be used to assess vertical dimension? What are their problems?*

Initially it is most straightforward to simply observe the vertical dimension with the denture removed (Fig. 15.1) and in place (Fig. 15.2).

Note the open lip posture (Fig. 15.2) when the denture is inserted. This is an important indicator that there may be an error in vertical height and a more accurate assessment must be made.

There are three common methods which might be used, the first two of which are essentially similar and suffer some of the same problems. These both measure the lower facial height at rest and with the dentures in occlusion. The difference between these measurements is the freeway space. The head must be in a natural vertical position supported by the neck muscles. A fixed support can alter the freeway space. In most instances these methods are satisfactory and readily applied, but sometimes it may be appropriate to use all three methods to establish the correct vertical dimension.

Dividers/callipers method. Marks or adhesive markers are placed on the chin and nose and their distance apart is measured with callipers or dividers. One problem is that the markers are fixed to the skin and may move through muscle activity, particularly pursing of the lips. All suitable sites on the skin may move to some degree so that it is necessary to check that the patient remains relaxed during the procedure.

This method is shown in Figures 15.1 and 15.2. The callipers are set to the resting face height (Fig. 15.1). When the denture is inserted (Fig. 15.2) the increase in vertical dimension is clearly seen and is about 3–4 mm.

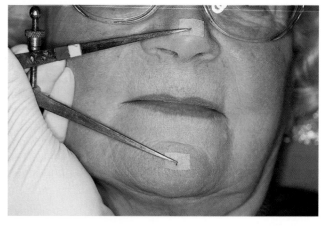
Fig. 15.1 Rest vertical dimension with the upper prosthesis removed.

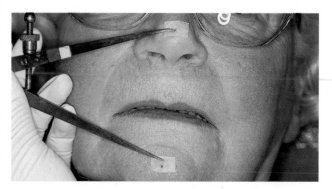
Fig. 15.2 Vertical dimension with the upper overdenture in place.

Willis bite gauge. This measures lower face height from the lower border of the nose and mandible. It is important to use the same pressure when recording rest and occlusal height; otherwise compression of the tissues will distort the reading. More importantly, the instrument has to be used at a consistent angle at the base of the nose. This is particularly difficult when making complete dentures against lower standing teeth, because removing the upper denture to record rest height removes the denture support of the upper lip which is used as a landmark.

Closed speaking space method. This method provides a rough estimate of the presence of a freeway space but does not involve direct measurement. The patient is asked to say words including prominent 'ss' sounds, such as 'Mississippi' and 'Tuesday'. These sounds are more difficult to make in the absence of freeway space. Unfortunately patients adapt their speech to both an increased or decreased occlusal height and this method can only be considered an adjunct to the more accurate methods above.

■ *How large should the freeway space be?*

This depends on the patient. The average freeway space is 2–4 mm measured in the premolar region, and dentures may be constructed to this dimension for most patients. However, there are some circumstances in which this clearance needs to be increased. Some patients become habituated to an increased freeway space, either because of worn artificial teeth or because of faulty denture construction. In some cases the freeway space may exceed a centimetre and it would be unreasonable to expect such patients to accommodate rapidly to the normal freeway space. Provided the increased freeway space is not associated with any problems a compromise increased freeway space is appropriate.

DIAGNOSIS

■ *What is your diagnosis and why is this the most likely possibility?*

Error in occlusal vertical dimension. There is clearly an increased occlusal vertical dimension, based on the measurements described above, and this is beyond the tolerance level of most patients. This fault is frequently associated with a history of being able to cope with the denture for a few hours and then having to remove the prosthesis. The open lip posture is also often associated with an increased occlusal vertical dimension. Some patients naturally have an open lip posture, so this sign is only an indication of potential problems. Until this fault is corrected, it is not really possible to consider any alternative explanation.

■ *What possible diagnoses have you excluded? Explain why for each possibility.*

Error in retruded position. Dentures with this fault produce pain on the ridge and pain on eating. If this were suspected it would be necessary to take a pre-contact occlusal check record and to remount the dentures on an articulator to make

a definitive diagnosis. Adjustment of the occlusion to the correct record should cure the symptoms and this will confirm the cause. This possible error needs to be kept in mind in all such cases. If the occlusion is ignored and the denture base adjusted, the area of soreness will move to another area with each adjustment, progressively destroying the fit surface of the denture.

Difficulty in becoming accustomed to acrylic palatal coverage. Three months is normally a sufficient time for a patient to become accustomed to a new denture design, even when there is a change to acrylic palatal coverage. In the very elderly, or those who have worn a denture for many years, this period may need to be extended, and a minority of patients need training bases or simple acrylic partial dentures before definitive complete dentures or overdentures. However, no patient should be expected to become accustomed to a denture with an increased vertical dimension.

Denture-related stomatitis. There was redness of the denture-bearing area and this almost certainly indicates denture stomatitis (chronic atrophic candidiasis). However, this condition is asymptomatic and not normally noticed by patients.

Patient's expectation of appearance has not been met. Both men and women may be embarrassed to admit that their dentures do not fulfil their cosmetic expectations. This may not just be the fault of the denture but also result from a patient's seeking to recapture their youthful appearance. While this may not be unreasonable, it may be physically impossible. Sometimes hurtful comments from relatives, friends or acquaintances may change the patient's opinion about an otherwise satisfactory denture. This problem may be manifest by repeated minor complaints that do not make sense clinically, or, as in this case, a dislike or complete rejection of the denture. This problem can only be diagnosed by careful and considerate questioning.

In the present case this possible diagnosis is unlikely given that there is a fault in the vertical dimension and the patient appears happy with the appearance of the denture.

Miscellaneous and other unusual complaints. These include complaints of irritation from a high residual monomer content in an incorrectly processed denture base, or the very rare hypersensitivity to acrylic. In both cases the denture-bearing area, and sometimes the whole mouth, would be sore. This patient has inflammation of the denture-bearing area but this is much more likely to be related to denture plaque or perhaps candidal infection and these should be excluded before considering the alternative causes. Another complaint sometimes unfairly ascribed to dentures is the symptom of mucosal burning in an otherwise healthy mouth. This is usually psychogenic and associated with depression. Nothing in the history suggests this diagnosis.

■ *How would you manage the case?*

Replace the missing restoration in the canine root to prevent caries.

To solve the denture problem, the denture must be remade with an appropriate freeway space, but first the denture stomatitis must be treated to improve support for the new prosthesis. A swab from the palate or fitting surface of the denture should be performed to detect candidal infection, unless the appearances are typical in which case treatment may be instituted immediately. Treatment will involve improving denture hygiene, ceasing night wear, if appropriate, and provision of a short course of antifungal treatment such as amphotericin lozenges (which must be sucked with the dentures removed from the mouth). The possibility of an underlying condition predisposing to candidiasis should be considered, especially if the infection involves other parts of the mouth or lips or if treatment fails despite good denture hygiene.

Summary

A 24-year-old gentleman is referred to you in your oral surgery-orientated practice for a second opinion on the need to remove his lower third molar teeth. Is this the correct decision, and if it is, how should it be achieved?

Complaint

The patient has no complaint at present but has been advised by his general dental practitioner to have his lower third molars extracted. He is very nervous about the extractions and requests a second opinion before deciding on treatment.

History of complaint

The patient has had two episodes of pericoronitis around the lower left third molar. The first was relatively mild but the second, about 3 months ago, was associated with inability to open the mouth and slight facial swelling and required a course of oral antibiotics.

Medical history

The patient is fit and well. He has had a general anaesthetic previously to reduce and fix a compound fracture of his arm which has been permanently plated. He has had no problems with bleeding following trauma.

EXAMINATION

Extraoral examination

The left submandibular lymph nodes are palpable but not tender. There is no facial asymmetry.

Intraoral examination

■ *What particular features of the intraoral examination are important and why?*

See Table 16.1.

In this case the patient has normal mouth opening, a full unrestored dentition without evidence of caries, periodontal disease or poor oral hygiene. The lower third molars are partially erupted and appear vertically orientated and there is mild inflammation of the attached gingivae surrounding both crowns. The upper third molars are overerupted and nonfunctional. The patient has a pronounced gag reflex when the teeth are examined.

INVESTIGATIONS

■ *Would you take radiographs? If so, which views would you take and why?*

Yes, radiographs are required to assess root morphology, degree of bone impaction, proximity to inferior dental nerve and the possibility of associated disease (for instance cysts, hypercementosis and temporomandibular joint problems).

The views to be possibly taken are listed, with their advantages and disadvantages, in Table 16.2.

Table 16.1 Important features of the intraoral examination

Feature	Reason
Interincisal opening	One feature determining access for surgical removal and affecting the difficulty of extraction. Trismus may also reflect infection or inflammation in the muscles of mastication.
Condition of rest of dentition	If the first or second molars have a poor prognosis through caries or are extensively restored, transplanting the third molars in their place might be considered.
Oral hygiene	Poor oral hygiene increases the risk of dry socket, soft tissue infection and delayed healing.
Position of lower third molars	The degree of eruption, angulation and proximity to the second molar are important. Partially erupted vertical or distoangular lower third molars are more at risk of pericoronitis than mesioangularly impacted ones.
Position of upper third molar	Nonfunctional upper third molars may overerupt and traumatize the operculum over the lower third molar or erupt buccally and traumatize the cheek. Both situations might contribute to symptoms.
Position of external oblique ridge	If this lies close behind or over the impacted tooth access is poor and considerable bone removal may be required if the tooth is large or impacted.
Condition of lower second molars	The lower second molar is at risk of iatrogenic damage during surgical removal of the third molar. Crowns or large restorations, especially those involving the distal surface, will be at risk and may increase the difficulty of the extraction.
Presence of pericoronitis	Has the same effect as generalized poor oral hygiene except that the risk of adverse effects is higher. Surgery should not be performed in an infected field.
Miscellaneous features	Factors such as a pronounced gag reflex, poor patient compliance and anxiety may all affect treatment.

Table 16.2 The radiographic views

View	Advantages	Disadvantages
Periapicals of upper and lower third molars	Provided the periapicals can be taken with a paralleling technique these are the ideal views. They provide a geometrically accurate projection with true relationships to the adjacent structures. They are also convenient for single extractions. These views are the first choice.	Unfortunately it may not be possible to obtain films using the paralleling technique because of patient tolerance. Placement of the film in the ideal position, showing the teeth and inferior dental nerve canal, is uncomfortable. If films are angled then a degree of distortion is inevitable.
Oblique laterals	Readily taken without specialized equipment. Show both upper and lower third molars without superimposition. Give a good view of the surrounding bone when adjacent lesions, e.g. cysts, are present. It is the second-best option.	Suffer a degree of distortion as the beam is angled upwards, so that the relationship to adjacent structures is not accurate.
Panoramic tomograph	Convenient survey film if equipment available. Gives a good view of the surrounding bone when adjacent lesions, e.g. cysts, are present. Though only third choice on technical merit, panoramic films are often used and in practice usually provide sufficient information to assess extractions.	Poor image quality because the view is a tomograph. In addition there is superimposition of the opposite angle of mandible over upper and lower third molars. The upward beam angle distorts the relationship between teeth and adjacent structures and the image is magnified. Root morphology often cannot be assessed on panoramic films.
Lower oblique occlusal	Useful when the lower third molar lies horizontally and is seen end-on in a periapical view. Provides information on buccolingual orientation. Useful if tooth lies out of the line of arch. Used only rarely.	

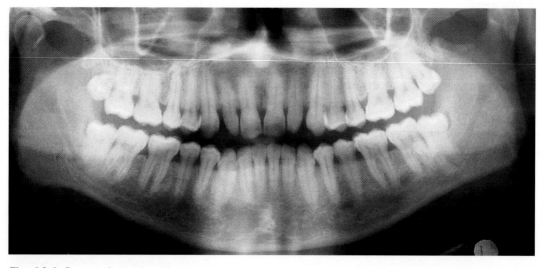

Fig. 16.1 Panoramic tomograph.

There is little to choose between these radiographic views in terms of radiation dose, provided fast films and appropriate intensifying screens are used.

In this case the patient's gag reflex prevented the taking of paralleling technique periapicals and so a panoramic tomograph was taken. It is shown in Figure 16.1.

■ *What does the radiograph show?*

The patient is fully dentate with no restoration or caries visible on the film. The lower third molars are vertically orientated and impacted against soft tissue rather than the second molars. The impacted teeth are of normal size and the surrounding bone appears to be of normal density. The roots of both teeth appear to be closely related to the inferior dental nerve canal,

there is darkening but no narrowing or deflection of the bony wall of the canal, suggesting that it does not contact or pass through the tooth root.

■ *You now have sufficient information to decide whether the third molars should be removed or not. What are the indications for removal?*

There has been much debate about indications for removal of third molars, and those for removal of asymptomatic third molars are particularly contentious. Mandibular impacted third molars (MITMs) are very common, affecting approximately 75% of 20–30-year-old patients. Surgery is unpleasant, carries risks and is expensive to state or patient; thus, following accepted guidelines is essential.

The suggested indications for removal are:
- Recurrent pericoronitis and pericoronitis with acute spreading infection.
- Unrestorable caries of MITM or adjacent teeth.
- Untreatable periapical inflammation.
- Periodontal disease associated with the MITM or adjacent teeth.
- Internal or external resorption of MITM or adjacent teeth.
- MITM in fracture line.
- Associated cysts or neoplasia.
- For tooth reimplantation.
- For orthognathic surgery or restorative treatment.
- Prophylactic removal may be advised in specific medical conditions.

■ *Should this patient's teeth be removed and why?*

Yes, he has suffered two episodes of pericoronitis. There is a greater risk of future episodes as the number of attacks increases, and they are likely to become more frequent and more severe.

■ *How will you decide whether extraction of this patient's third molars is within your ability?*

Easier extraction	More difficult extraction
Young patient	Patient aged over 30
Female patient	Male patient
Caucasoid/Mongoloid racial stock	Negroid racial stock
Superficial impaction	Deeply buried
Mesioangular or vertical impaction	Distoangular or horizontal impaction
Small crown	Wide crown
Conical root	Multirooted, divergent roots
Lying buccally in relation to line of arch	Lying lingually in relation to line of arch
Clear path of delivery, usually forward and upward	Vertical or distal path of removal required, possibly requiring tooth section
External oblique ridge well posterior to tooth	External oblique ridge overlies tooth
Sound second molar	Crowned, root-treated or heavily restored adjacent molar
Normal second molar root morphology	Conical root (risks accidental elevation)
Distant from ID nerve	Adjacent to ID nerve
Large dental follicle	Narrow dental follicle or ankylosis
Good access	Poor access, trismus
Not impacted or soft tissue impacted	Impacted against bone or root of second molar
	History of complex or difficult extraction

This is a matter of judgement. You must judge your own ability and experience against the likely difficulty and also consider your ability to manage any complications. In general the following factors should be considered:
The most important of these factors may be remembered using the mnemonic WHARFE:

W angulation using **W**inter's lines
H **H**eight of mandible
A **A**ngle of second molar
R **R**oot form and development
F size of **F**ollicular sac
E **E**xit path of tooth to be extracted

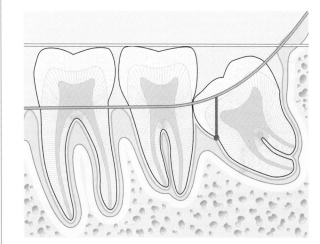

Fig. 16.2 Example of the application of Winter's lines.

■ *What are 'Winter's lines' and how might they help assess difficulty?*

To apply Winter's lines, three imaginary lines are drawn on the radiographic image (Fig. 16.2). For descriptive purposes the lines are assigned colours. The white line runs along the occlusal plane, and the amber line runs along the upper bone surface through the interdental bone crests and along the bone surface behind the third molar (not up the external oblique ridge). The red line passes vertically, at right angles to the white line to the application point for an elevator. In mesioangular impactions the point of elevation lies at the mesial end of the amelocemental junction, and for distoangular impactions it lies at the distal end of the amelocemental junction.

The angle of impaction is judged against the white line. The amber line gives an indication of the amount of tooth which will be visible when the periosteal flap is raised and the amount of bone removal required over the crown. The red line gives an indication of the depth of bone removal required to gain a point of application for an elevator. If the red line is more than 5 mm in length the extraction is likely to merit general anaesthetic. If it is greater than 9 mm, it is likely that extensive bone removal will be required.

■ *What are the deficiencies of the Winter's lines technique?*

Winter's lines are useful for mesioangular impactions but the length of the red line is almost meaningless in distoangular impactions. The technique also ignores the possibility of sectioning the tooth which makes the extraction easier, changing the point of application of elevators and the path of removal. Winter's lines should be applied to a periapical radiograph, preferably a geometrically accurate projection obtained by a paralleling technique. The method can be used on oblique laterals or panoramic tomographs but then provides a less accurate estimate of difficulty. In addition, a correction must be made for magnification in the panoral film, which ranges from × 1.2 to × 1.4 depending on the equipment used.

Winter's lines would not provide useful information in the present case, but they do provide a way of systematically examining a radiograph to ensure that no information is missed.

■ *How difficult are this patient's extractions?*

Both lower third molars are slightly distoangularly inclined and the external oblique ridge overlies them. Though not very deeply placed these are moderately difficult extractions which should not be tackled under local anaesthetic other than by an experienced or specialized surgeon. Extraction of these teeth is not appropriate in the general practice setting.

The majority of lower third molars which meet the criteria for extraction (listed above) will be relatively difficult. This is because the commonest indication is pericoronitis which affects mostly vertically and distoangularly impacted teeth.

■ *Prior to surgery you must warn the patient about the complications of removal. List the possible complications and give an indication of their frequency.*

See Table 16.3.

■ *What warnings would you give to the patient about extraction?*

Deciding exactly which complications to warn patients about can be difficult. The decision must be made for each case. The patient must be provided with sufficient information to give informed consent and the clinician must answer all the patient's questions correctly. It is generally considered mandatory to warn the patient about both sequelae and the significant complications. Sequelae may be induced by surgery or anaesthetic and should be differentiated. Surgical sequelae include swelling (for 48 hours), pain (for approximately 48 hours), bleeding (for about 2 hours), sore temporomandibular joint and trismus, sensitivity of the adjacent teeth, and remodelling of the sockets for approximately 10–12 weeks. Complications which must be described are the risk of dry socket and the risk of temporary and permanent damage to lingual and inferior dental nerves. Warnings concerning damage to adjacent teeth or restorations, or displacement of teeth into the antrum, are usually reserved for patients who are at particular risk.

Table 16.3 Possible complications of removal

Complication	Frequency
Postsurgical pain, haemorrhage, trismus, swelling and ecchymosis	These affect all patients to some degree and in a proportion of cases may be prolonged. Inability to eat and enjoy food is considered a significant complication by patients.
Alveolar osteitis (dry socket)	Affects 1–35% lower third molar extractions, depending on difficulty and technique.
Sensory nerve damage, paraesthesia or anaesthesia	Affects 10–20% of cases though almost all recover spontaneously. A degree of permanent damage to inferior dental or lingual nerves affects 0.5% of cases.
Acute temporomandibular joint pain/ dysfunction (myofascial pain syndrome).	About 4% of cases, higher in patients with pre-existing symptoms and those whose teeth are removed under general anaesthesia. A mild degree of muscle and joint discomfort is probably much commoner.
Iatrogenic fracture	Fracture of the mandible is fortunately rare, occurring in 1 per 10 000 cases. If minor fractures of the alveolar or lingual plates or tuberosity are included, the incidence is 2–4% of cases, but apart from tuberosity fracture these are mostly of little consequence.
Incorrect or incomplete extraction	Less than 1%
Acute/chronic postoperative infection including osteonecrosis	Rare, affecting 2–3 per 100 000 cases.
Injury to adjacent structures including teeth and periodontium	Not uncommon; occurs in 3 per 1000 cases.
Oroantral fistula	Rare.
Introduction of tooth or fragment into another tissue space (antrum, tissue space, inhaled into lung or swallowed)	Rare.
Systemic medical/surgical complications related to surgery and/or anaesthetic	Sore throat, adverse reaction, etc. Patients must not drive or operate machinery for 48 hours after sedation or general anaesthesia.
Death under outpatient general anaesthetic	1 per 200 000. Increased risk in children. May be related to Halothane induced cardiac arrhythmias.

■ *Does the patient require antibiotic cover before surgery to prevent infection of the bone plate in his arm?*

No, this is not necessary.

■ *Would you prescribe postoperative antibiotics for these extractions?*

There are no universally agreed criteria for providing antibiotics postoperatively. Antibiotics do not affect the incidence of dry socket and should not be given without reason. They would be indicated if there were an increased risk of infection, as in a diabetic or immunosuppressed patient, or if infection were present at the time of operation. However, in normal

individuals, antibiotics are probably less important than local measures for preventing infection. A chlorhexidine mouthrinse before operation and/or debridement of the teeth and below the operculum are highly effective in reducing the incidence of postoperative infection and the bacteraemia which may lead to endocarditis.

In some centres antibiotics are given routinely whenever bone removal is required. In others none are given and their value is disputed. If antibiotics are provided, patients having extractions under local anaesthesia usually receive an oral course of amoxicillin or metronidazole. When general anaesthesia is used, a suitable regime would be a single intravenous bolus dose of 750 mg cefuroxime.

Osteomyelitis is a particular problem because it can be difficult to treat effectively. All those at increased risk should

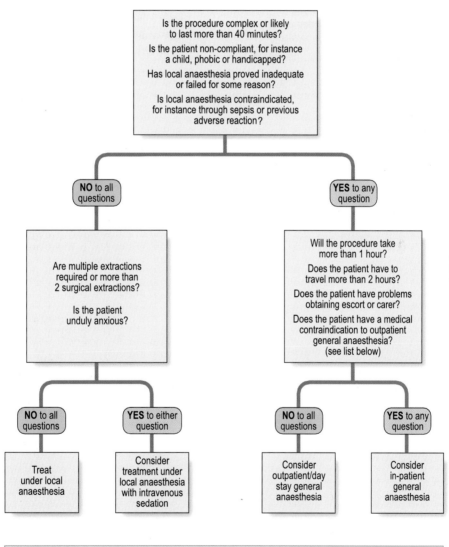

Fig. 16.3 Flow chart for selection of patients for general anaesthesia.

receive antibiotics. Examples are patients in whom bone is sclerotic or has a reduced blood supply, for instance after radiotherapy involving the jaws or when large periosteal flaps are raised in the very elderly. Larger doses than normal and longer courses may be provided.

■ *Is a general anaesthetic required or desirable?*

The choice of anaesthetic will depend on the indications for treatment, the assessment of difficulty and the anaesthetic risk assessment for the particular patient.

This patient requires extraction of all four third molars. The indications for removal do not in themselves require a general anaesthetic. However, the surgery is likely to take longer than 20 minutes on each side under local anaesthetic. Arguably this procedure could be performed under local anaesthesia in two visits by an experienced clinician but many patients find this unacceptable. The patient's gag reflex is one factor suggesting that general anaesthesia or sedation would be appropriate, and the patient appears to have no medical contraindication. The patient must be fully informed of the risks of sedation or anaesthesia before making a decision. The risks of general anaesthesia are such that it is never the anaesthetic of choice for routine or straightforward extractions. The flow chart (Fig. 16.3) illustrates some factors in selecting a suitable anaesthetic.

■ *What surgical technique should be used to remove the lower third molars?*

There is much debate about the best method for removal of lower third molars. Some authorities suggests that the buccal technique should become the accepted method. In this system no lingual flap is raised and no lingual nerve retraction is performed so that this method carries a minimal risk of permanent nerve damage. Although this is the standard method used in Europe and the USA, in the UK it has been traditional to raise lingual and buccal flaps. Under local anaesthetic it is usual to remove bone buccally with a bur, while under general anaesthetic the lingual plate is removed with a chisel using the lingual split technique.

CASE 17 Discoloured anterior teeth

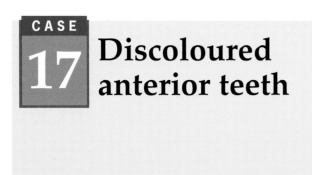

Summary

A 22-year-old woman presents at your general dental practice surgery complaining of the poor appearance of her teeth. What is the cause and what treatment is appropriate?

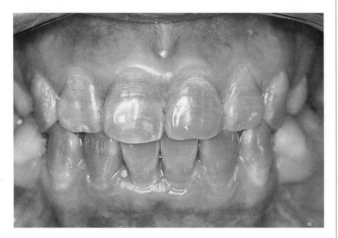

Fig. 17.1 The appearance of the teeth.

HISTORY

Complaint

She is unhappy with the colour of the teeth which she feels are becoming darker. She is very conscious of them and realizes that she is reluctant to smile because of their appearance.

History of complaint

The teeth looked grey on eruption but they have slowly darkened.

Dental history

The patient has had very little dental treatment but received regular preventive care from your practice until the age of 16. Your notes record that she was given oral fluoride supplementation as a child. This was provided as fluoride drops at a dose of 0.25 mg daily from birth to 2 years and 0.5 mg daily as tablets from 2 to 4 years, rising to 1 mg daily from 4 to 12 years of age.

Medical history

The patient is fit and healthy with no relevant medical conditions noted on her medical history questionnaire.

■ *What are the possible causes of discolouration of teeth? What features of each cause aid differential diagnosis?*

The possible causes and relevant features are presented in Table 17.1.

■ *What specific questions would you ask this patient? Explain why.*

Did she suffer any illness between birth and 6 years? This might account directly for the discolouration or could have been the cause of antibiotic treatment with tetracyclines. Further information on chronological hypoplasia will be found in Case 37.

What toothpaste was used during fluoride supplementation? The fluoride supplementation regime provided for this patient was recommended during her childhood, but the doses would now be considered too high. On these doses, a small proportion of patients would be expected to show mild fluorosis. More severe fluorosis would be associated with a second source of fluoride. The most probable additional source would be ingestion of adult-formula fluoride toothpaste, though living in an area with fluoridated water should also be excluded.

Is there a family history of tooth discolouration or tooth loss? A positive family history aids diagnosis of inherited defects and is essential for diagnosis of some types of amelogenesis imperfecta.

In response to your questioning the patient tells you that she remembers taking many courses of antibiotics as a child for chest infections. She cannot remember what toothpaste she used before the age of 6, but for as long as she can remember she has used an adult paste. She has no family history of similar defects.

EXAMINATION

Intraoral examination

On examination the oral mucosa is healthy and oral hygiene is good. The dentition is unrestored.

■ *The appearance of the anterior teeth is shown in Figure 17.1. What do you see? How do you interpret the appearance?*

The morphology of the tooth crowns is normal and the incisors, canines and premolars are a grey-brown colour. There are some areas which appear less affected and others which appear opaque white. Small flecks of white are scattered on the labial enamel. There are several prominent horizontal lines on the teeth, most clearly seen in the enamel of the gingival third of the crowns of both upper central incisors.

The teeth are evenly discoloured and this has the appearance of an intrinsic stain. The distribution of the affected enamel is in a chronological pattern and affects all enamel formed from birth to approximately 6 years of age. The even distribution suggests that the cause was present

Table 17.1 Possible causes of discolouration

Causes	Features
Extrinsic staining	
Dietary stains such as tea, coffee, cigarette smoke, betel quid Chlorhexidine mouthwash Pigments produced by the normal oral flora, usually the subgingival flora	Usually worse around gingival margin and in less well cleaned areas because these agents stain pellicle and plaque rather than enamel.
Turner tooth	Infection of the deciduous predecessor causes enamel hypoplasia in a permanent tooth and the porous enamel absorbs extrinsic stains. Tooth shape abnormal.
Intrinsic staining	
Dental caries	Associated with softening. Characteristic distribution of lesions. Slowly progressing and dentine caries are the types most frequently stained.
Blood pigments	Seen most frequently in nonvital teeth (as a result of pulp necrosis). Rarely may affect all teeth in conditions including rhesus incompatibility (in the deciduous teeth only), porphyria and hyperbilirubinaemia. Colour ranges from dull red through brown to grey or black.
Tetracycline staining	Caused by administration of tetracyclines during tooth formation. When severe, this is a generalized green, brown or yellow colour, darkening with time. The teeth may fluoresce under ultraviolet light in the early stages but this reduces as the colour darkens. When mild there may be a chronological banding pattern with horizontal lines of discoloured enamel corresponding to individual courses of tetracycline. Tooth shape is normal.
Fluorosis	Varies from mild flecks of opaque white enamel to severely hypoplastic patches which take up extrinsic stain. The latter is only seen in areas where fluorosis is endemic. The mildest effects are impossible to tell from the opaque flecks seen when water fluoride concentration is very low. Affects all teeth. Moderately affected cases of endemic fluorosis may have an apparent chronological pattern of fine white lines associated with periods of exposure to higher doses. Tooth shape normal unless condition is severe.
Amelogenesis imperfecta	Numerous types. Affects all teeth, though some forms are much milder in the deciduous dentition. Colour change varies and is secondary to either hypoplasia (thin hard translucent enamel through which dentine is visible), hypocalcification (chalky white opaque soft enamel) and hypomaturation (patchy distribution of white opacities). Affected areas may also take up extrinsic stain. Tooth shape may be normal and some types have a vertical banding, pitting or ridging pattern. Family history will be positive in most cases. Mild types are difficult to distinguish from fluorosis.
Dentinogenesis imperfecta	All teeth are an even grey-brown colour with altered translucency. The shape of the tooth crowns is normal but the roots are thin and taper sharply. There is gradual pulpal obliteration by dentine. There may be a family history and, in some cases, osteogenesis imperfecta is associated. Enamel fractures from the dentine and severe wear follows shortly after eruption.
Regional odontodysplasia	Affects a group of adjacent deciduous and permanent teeth on one side of midline. Enamel hypoplasia leads to uptake of extrinsic stain and yellow cementum may be present over the crown. Characteristic defects on radiography include thin enamel and dentine, large pulps. Affected teeth often fail to erupt.
Chronological hypoplasia	Horizontal band(s) of enamel hypoplasia, each associated with a specific insult, usually a severe illness or metabolic upset including severe attacks of the common viral diseases of childhood. Affected bands are abnormal enamel which may be pitted, hypoplastic, rough, opaque or completely absent, and also take up extrinsic stain.
Age change	Teeth become yellower and slightly darker with age. This is an even colour change and it is usually mild.

throughout development or that there were frequent or prolonged exposures. The fine lines in the central incisors suggest that a series of repeated exposures is the more likely cause. The grey-brown colour is typical of tetracycline staining.

The small white flecks are more difficult to explain. They are not consistent with tetracycline staining and could be either mild fluorosis or a normal feature made more prominent by the dark enamel.

INVESTIGATION

■ *What further examinations would you carry out? Explain why.*

The teeth should be examined after drying. This makes porous defects more opaque and more visible and aids the detection of fine chronological bands and enamel flecks. The teeth could also be examined under an ultraviolet (UV) light or near UV light to see whether they fluoresce green/yellow because this would indicate tetracycline staining. The fluorescence is not bright and cannot be seen unless the room is dark and the illuminating lamp has a very low visible light output.

Though not necessary for diagnosis in this case, it is always prudent to test the vitality of discoloured teeth in case loss of vitality is the cause. The vitality of the affected teeth would determine the treatment options available.

Radiography is not a useful investigation in the present case. Periapical radiographs would be indicated if teeth were nonvital or affected by periodontitis. They would also be helpful in a younger patient to determine whether unerupted teeth were normal or if dentinogenesis imperfecta were considered a likely cause.

In this case no fluorescence could be detected in the surgery and all teeth were vital.

DIFFERENTIAL DIAGNOSIS

■ *What is your diagnosis?*

The dark colour of the teeth is typical of intrinsic staining caused by tetracycline. The history of yellow teeth becoming darker over a period of years is also characteristic.

An enquiry to the patient's medical practitioner confirms that as a child she received repeated and sometimes prolonged courses of tetracycline for chest infection, confirming the diagnosis.

■ *Why is fluorosis not the cause?*

Fluorosis cannot account for the generalized discolouration. The appearances are quite different, with mottled brown and white patches. The scattered white flecks could be caused by mild fluorosis and the fact that the patient used a fluoride toothpaste as well as a fluoride supplement for many years makes this a possibility. However, no definitive diagnosis can be reached because there is no accepted diagnostic test for mild degrees of fluorosis. Small numbers of such small white flecks are found in normal enamel.

TREATMENT

■ *How would you decide which teeth should be treated?*

The patient's main concern is her appearance. Only those teeth which are affected and visible need be treated. The factors which should be taken into account are the following.

The smile line. Observe the patient relaxed, talking and smiling naturally. Note the level of the lip line, which teeth and how much of each crown is visible. This will dictate which teeth need treatment and, if restorations are necessary, where the cervical margin should be placed. In this case all upper teeth from first molar to first molar are visible during smiling but second premolars and molars lie in shadow and the staining is not obvious. The upper lip line runs along the gingival margin of all upper incisors and canines, exposing the interdental papillae.

The occlusion. Indirect porcelain or composite veneers are difficult to make where the teeth are imbricated because the teeth on the die model cannot be separated in the laboratory. Alternative methods of treatment must be used. If there is wear on the incisal edge then porcelain veneers, which are inherently brittle, may fracture and direct composite veneers may be preferable.

Occupation. A patient whose occupation depends on their appearance may require both a greater degree of correction of the tooth shade and treatment of a larger number of tooth surfaces. Performers and others who work in bright, even artificial light may also require restorations to look natural under demanding lighting conditions. Fortunately, these more unusual constraints do not apply to this patient.

■ *What treatment options are available? What are their advantages and disadvantages?*

The treatment options are presented in Table 17.2.

Table 17.2 Treatment options

Option	Advantages	Disadvantages
Vital bleaching agents using carbamide (or urea) peroxide	Work best with extrinsic stains and quite well for many intrinsic stains. Easily applied in custom trays, nondestructive and easily repeated if necessary. Does not alter the underlying tooth shade or translucency. If sufficient and even lightening of the shade is achieved, bleaching produces the best appearance of all options. Can also be used to mask severe staining before a veneer is placed. This prevents the dark enamel showing through and allows a more translucent veneer to be used, improving the final appearance.	Unpredictable effectiveness with tetracycline staining, often leaving a dark zone cervically where the stained root shows through the thin cervical enamel. However, almost always some improvement and this may satisfy the patient. Only appropriate when there are minimal or no restorations in the teeth. Restorations are not bleached and there is a theoretical concern that bleaching agents might track to the pulp along the margins of restorations. Some over-the-counter formulations are acidic and others may cause local soft tissue irritation, and should not be encouraged. Licensing regulations vary between countries.
Nonvital bleach	Allows bleaching of deeper dentine than a vital bleach, producing greater effect.	Only possible in nonvital teeth and so usually inappropriate for multiple teeth. To bleach dentine below the cervical enamel the bleaching agent must be applied to the cervical part of the root canal as well as the pulp chamber.

Table 17.2 *Cont'd*

Option	Advantages	Disadvantages
Direct composite, indirect composite or porcelain veneers	Good appearance possible, can be as good as crowns but much less destructive.	Some tooth preparation is required, the amount varying slightly between types. The 'emergence profile' or contour at the gingival margin must be maintained by removing cervical enamel, to avoid a plaque trap. When placed over darkly stained teeth, veneer and cement must be opaque. This reduces translucency and produces a 'flat' artificial colour to the finished restoration. Expensive.
Crowns	Strong and retentive, a variety of bonded or reinforced crowns are available if the occlusion is a problem. Very darkly stained teeth are best crowned. The porcelain is thicker than veneers so that opaque materials are not required. If necessary, metal-bonded crowns completely mask the underlying colour. Usually the best alternative if the teeth contain extensive restorations. Appearance can be excellent.	Destructive of tooth tissue. Margins may compromise periodontal health. Expensive

■ *Which treatment is appropriate for this patient? Explain why.*

The selection of appropriate treatment is outlined in the flow chart (Figure 17.3, p. 75).

A conservative approach using carbamide peroxide bleaching agents would be appropriate initially. However, in this case the patient's lip line leaves the cervical enamel of the incisors and canines exposed and the effectiveness of the result is not predictable. Dark stain remained cervically after bleaching and the patient requested porcelain veneers to mask the discolouration.

PROGNOSIS

The completed porcelain veneers are shown in Figure 17.2. The appearance is not ideal and the disadvantage of having to use opaque veneers is well shown. However, the patient was very happy with this result.

■ *What is the long-term prognosis for these veneers?*

The veneers on the upper right canine and lateral incisor are in crossbite with the lower canine and almost edge to edge on the lateral incisor. On the upper left the same teeth are edge to edge. There is a risk of chipping the incisal edges and debonding.

PREVENTION

■ *Tetracycline should no longer be prescribed to those below the age of 12. Presumably tetracycline staining should no longer be seen?*

This is true, but unfortunately courses of tetracycline are still occasionally prescribed for children. There are some specific indications, such as cystic fibrosis, for which prolonged tetracycline treatment is still provided to children. Tetracyclines are available as over-the-counter drugs in some countries.

Tetracyclines such as minocycline, which are well absorbed and reach high blood levels, are the drugs of choice to prevent infection in acne. They are frequently prescribed to adolescents and young adults and may stain dental tissues forming at this time, such as the roots of third molars. However, minocycline may also stain bone and fully formed teeth. The drug becomes incorporated into the pulpal surface of the dentine and staining is darkest in teeth where there is active secondary dentine formation. Because this stain lies deep in the tooth, it cannot be bleached by external bleaching agents.

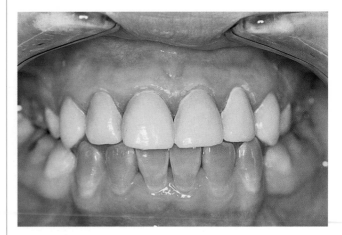

Fig. 17.2 The completed porcelain veneers immediately after cementation.

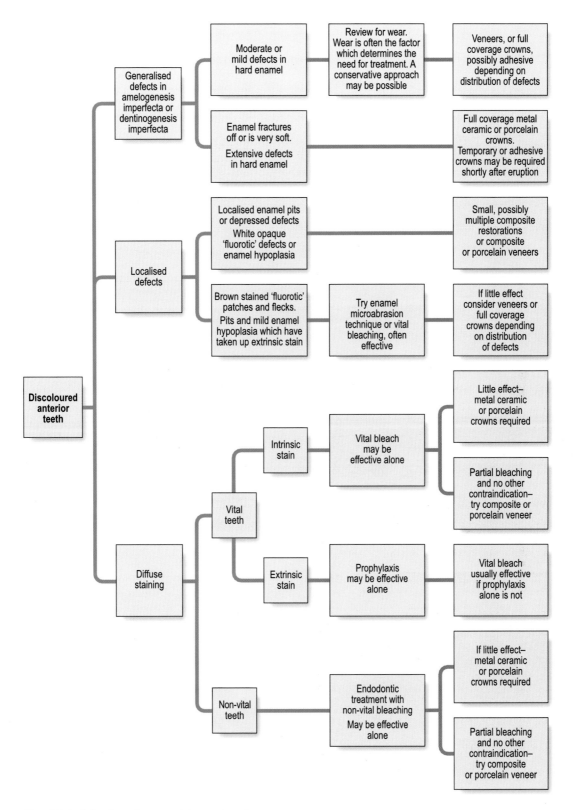

Fig. 17.3 Selection of appropriate treatment.

CASE
18 A very painful mouth

Summary

A 20-year-old man presents to you in your general dental practice, feeling ill and with a very sore mouth.

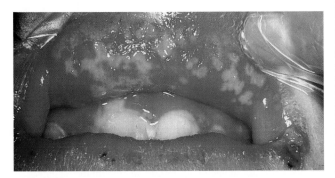

Fig. 18.1 Appearance of the patient's mouth.

HISTORY

Complaint

The patient complains of pain which is preventing eating and hampering drinking. He also feels unwell.

History of complaint

He first noticed feeling unwell 4 days previously and thought he had 'flu. He was slightly feverish and developed a headache. His mouth was sore but it was not until about 1 day later that it became very painful. Because he felt unable to take time off work, he took the remains of a course of an unknown oral antibiotic which had been prescribed for his brother who had an infected cut on his arm. This did not appear to have led to any improvement. He has had no similar attacks before.

Medical history

The patient is otherwise fit and well.

EXAMINATION

Extraoral examination

The patient has enlarged cervical lymph nodes which are slightly tender, mobile but soft or firm rather than hard. Apart from this finding no abnormalities are found in a routine examination of the head, neck and hands.

Intraoral examination

■ *What do you see in Figure 18.1?*

There are numerous ulcers on the labial mucosa which have the following characteristics:

Site	Labial mucosa and attached gingiva
Size	A few millimetres in diameter
Shape	Well defined, rounded, sometimes coalescing to form larger irregular ulcers
Colour	Covered by a yellow-grey fibrin ulcer slough, no well defined rim of periulcer erythema
Background	The surrounding mucosa appears uniformly inflamed

In addition, one large ulcer lies at the commissure and there are small bloodstained crusts around the lips.

If you were able to examine the patient you would discover that more ulcers affect much of the oral mucosa, including the gingivae, palate and tongue, and that they extend back into the oropharynx.

■ *Give a differential diagnosis on the basis of the information you have so far.*

- Primary herpetic gingivostomatitis
- Erythema multiforme.

■ *Justify this differential diagnosis.*

Primary herpetic gingivostomatitis and other oral viral infections typically cause multiple round small ulcers of acute onset, sometimes coalescing, on a background of inflamed mucosa. The patient feels unwell and has enlarged tender lymph nodes suggesting infection. Primary *Herpes simplex* infection usually affects much of the mucosa and has a predilection for the keratinized masticatory mucosa of the gingiva. The patient is older than is normally expected for a primary infection. However, the average age of patients with this infection has increased over the last few decades because improved living conditions have resulted in fewer individuals coming into contact with the virus.

Erythema multiforme (Stevens–Johnson syndrome) is possible. The acute onset and bloody crusts on the lips suggest this diagnosis and the age of the patient is compatible. However, the distribution of ulcers is not particularly suggestive of this condition. Erythema multiforme usually primarily affects the lips and nonkeratinized lining mucosa of the anterior mouth, and the ulcers have ragged margins, whereas the irregular ulcers in the picture seem to be formed by coalescence of small round ulcers. A trigger for erythema multiforme is sometimes identified and antibiotics, particularly sulphonamides, are sometimes the cause. This patient has had recent antibiotics but only after the symptoms appeared. Erythema multiforme is typically recurrent and the history of previous attacks and their periodicity is important in making the diagnosis. However, in a first attack the features may be milder and, as in this case, there is no history of similar attacks.

■ *What diagnoses have you discounted and why?*

Other oral viral infections do not produce a clinical picture of this severity. Herpangina and hand, foot and mouth disease are milder and usually affect the soft palate of children. *Varicella zoster* would be expected to cause chicken pox in this age group though children are the age group more typically affected; oral zoster in older patients is unilateral.

Herpetiform aphthae should be considered but are readily excluded. The ulcers may be numerous, small and coalescing and may have an erythematous background. However they are usually limited to the anterior or posterior of the mouth, do not affect keratinized mucosa and are not accompanied by systemic illness. Attacks are recurrent.

In a mild primary attack of *Herpes simplex* infection in an adult, the ulcers may be limited to the gingiva, raising the possibility of acute necrotizing ulcerative gingivitis. However, in this case the ulceration is too extensive for necrotizing gingivitis to be considered, and it is, in any case usually clinically characteristic.

■ *What further questions would you ask and what further examinations would you perform and why?*

Do you suffer from 'cold sores'? If the patient has had recurrent *Herpes simplex* infection, usually in the form of herpes labialis before, then the present ulcers cannot be due to a primary herpetic infection. Recurrent herpetic infection is sometimes a trigger for attacks of erythema multiforme and a cold sore 1–2 weeks before onset would raise this possibility.

In answer to this question, the patient indicates that he does not suffer from cold sores.

Have you been in contact with anyone with cold sores? Identification of a possible source of *Herpes simplex* 1–2 weeks before the ulcers would give further credibility to this diagnosis. Contact with *Herpes zoster* is not significant in this case but in less clear-cut cases it would be prudent to ask about chicken pox and shingles contacts.

The patient has no known contact with any viral disease.

Did you notice small blisters in your mouth before the ulcers appeared? This would suggest herpes virus infection, each ulcer being preceded by a small round vesicle. Larger vesicles and blisters are also found in erythema multiforme but these are irregular and usually limited to the vermilion border of the lips and floor of mouth.

Have you taken any drugs or medicines in the last 3 weeks? This will clarify the possibility that medication has triggered an attack of erythema multiforme.

The patient has taken no medication apart from the antibiotic noted in the history.

Have you any rash anywhere on your body? Erythema multiforme is associated with a variety of rashes (hence its name) and the patient should have a skin examination. The presence of typical target lesions indicates erythema multiforme but other less characteristic rashes should also be noted, together with their time of onset.

No rash is present.

Take the patient's temperature. This simple investigation is easily forgotten, but often valuable. A raised temperature in the early stages indicates infection. The temperature is not raised in erythema multiforme even when severe (unless there is infection of skin lesions).

His temperature is 38°C.

DIAGNOSIS

This differential diagnosis sometimes poses problems. If the patient has erythema multiforme he should be treated with a moderately high dose of systemic steroids, but this should be avoided if he has a viral infection. A period of time must elapse before the results of investigations will be available.

■ *Can you make a diagnosis and commence treatment?*

Yes. In this particular case there is sufficient evidence to make a working diagnosis of primary *Herpes simplex* infection. Investigations should be performed to confirm the diagnosis but need not delay treatment. Investigations are probably only available to those in hospital practice. Practitioners confident in the diagnosis might well instigate treatment without confirmatory tests.

INVESTIGATIONS

■ *What investigations might you consider, and what are their advantages and disadvantages?*

See Table 18.1.

In the current case, a smear for light microscopy and viral antibody titre against *Herpes simplex* were requested.

TREATMENT

■ *What treatment would you provide?*

The patient should be reassured that he has a common viral infection which, while unpleasant, has no significant implications. It will run its course in a further 10 days or so but it is unlikely to worsen significantly now that it is in its fifth day. Some adult patients may confuse this diagnosis with genital herpes and require some additional explanation.

While unwell the patient should rest and maintain a good fluid intake. This is especially important in children who refuse fluids and become dehydrated rapidly. A sedative antihistamine such as promethazine is sometimes suggested for very small and fractious children who cannot sleep during the acute phase. It also has the advantage of drying the reflex salivation.

Table 18.1 Investigations to be considered

Test	Advantages and disadvantages
Smear for light microscopy	Simple and rapid. Characteristic viral changes may indicate herpes virus infection provided epithelial cells from the ulcer margin are present in the smear. Most hospitals should be able to give an urgent result the same day. However, a smear will only be positive for the first few days of ulceration. As a result, a positive smear indicates infection but a negative smear cannot exclude it in all cases.
Swab for viral culture	Simple but takes several days. In general terms this test has the advantage that it detects a wide range of viruses but in this differential diagnosis the broad specificity is not particularly helpful.
Swab for viral antigen screen	Simple and moderately fast. A small number of viruses may be identified from their antigens in a swab using ELISA (enzyme-linked immunosorbent assay). Results from this test may be available in 24 hours but it is only available in some centres.
Swab for polymerase chain reaction (PCR)-based viral detection	Obtaining the smear is simple but the laboratory procedure is complex. Highly specific and moderately fast. Results should be available in 24–48 hours. The test is only available in specialized centres.
Smear for electron microscopy	Very specific and relatively simple but again only available in specialized centres. The result is usually available the same day.
Serum for viral antibody level	Serum for antibody to herpes and other viruses is simple to obtain and provides a result in about 48 hours. A high titre of IgM indicates acute infection (though it may take a day or two to rise to a detectable level) and IgG denotes a previous infection. In the absence of raised IgM, two samples several days apart to demonstrate an increasing IgG level are required for confident diagnosis of primary infection. This test is widely available and frequently used.
Biopsy of ulcer	Relatively readily performed but almost never necessary in *Herpes simplex* infection (except for the unusual chronic infections found in the immunosuppressed). Will give the diagnosis of herpetic infection in almost all cases. Also diagnostic in most cases of erythema multiforme.

The patient should be warned about infectivity. The virus is transmitted only by close contact but while there are vesicles or ulcers in the mouth, the saliva is infectious. Care should be taken to avoid close contact with other individuals, especially children. In the non-immune patient (by definition a person with a primary infection) other sites may also become infected and particular care should be taken not to spread saliva to the eye.

Antiviral treatment with aciclovir should be considered. Aciclovir is only effective in the earliest stage of the infection when virus is replicating. It must be taken in the first 48 hours for best effect, while vesicles rather than ulcers are present. Aciclovir is not indicated in this case because of the delay in presentation (though it might be considered in an immunosuppressed patient). A dose of 200 mg 5 times daily is recommended for immunocompetent patients. Related drugs giving higher levels in the blood, such as valaciclovir, are usually reserved for *Varicella zoster* infection.

Preparations for symptomatic relief of the oral ulceration are indicated. Tetracycline mouthwash (250 mg capsule of a soluble preparation dissolved in water, used 4 times daily) is very useful in reducing discomfort and would be an appropriate choice in this patient who has presented too late to benefit from aciclovir. Antiseptic mouthwashes such as chlorhexidine are also effective. These presumably reduce oral discomfort by preventing bacterial infection of the ulcers. Chlorhexidine would also compensate for difficulty in carrying out oral hygiene procedures. Analgesic mouthwashes such as benzydamine are an alternative.

PROGNOSIS

■ *What is the risk that this patient will suffer from cold sores in the future?*

Between 15 and 30% of individuals who come into contact with the virus develop recurrent infection. It is not clear whether those who suffer a symptomatic primary infection such as gingivostomatitis have an increased risk. Although this percentage seems high, many patients with recurrent herpes infection suffer only very occasional lesions.

■ *When would you ask the patient to return?*

The patient should return in about 1 week to check that healing is progressing, but earlier if symptoms worsen or new signs develop.

At some stage during treatment or follow up the patient should be warned not to take medications prescribed for others. The patient's brother's antibiotic was apparently a harmless but inappropriate drug. Those who take others' drugs run the risk of hypersensitivity, drug interaction or other unwanted reaction. The importance of completing the prescribed dose should be emphasized to all patients receiving antibiotics, both to ensure effective treatment and because this is critically important in preventing the emergence of resistant strains in the community.

FINAL OUTCOME

The next day a report on the smear for microscopy shows no evidence of viral infection (possibly because the ulcers have been present for several days), but on the following day the serum antibody result by complement fixation test shows an anti-*Herpes simplex* type 1 antibody titre of 160 (normal < 10). The diagnosis of herpetic gingivostomatitis is confirmed.

Radiographic errors

19

Summary

The figures show intraoral radiographs. Each one has been rejected as being diagnostically unacceptable. What is wrong with each and what are the possible explanations?

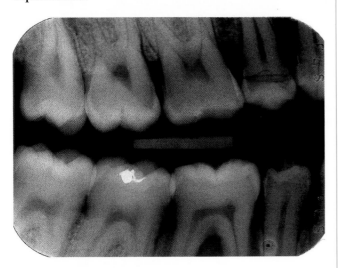

Fig. 19.1 A bitewing film.

■ *What is wrong with the film?*

The film is too dark. There is contrast between enamel and dentine but it is not possible to detect the subtler features of the teeth or to see the margin or internal structure in the alveolar bone.

■ *How might this error have been caused?*

The film can be too dark for three reasons, each of which has a number of possible explanations:

Reason	Possible causes
Overexposure	Usually the time of the exposure is too great because the incorrect exposure setting has been selected by the operator.
	The X-ray set timer may be faulty.
Overdevelopment	The developer solution could be too hot or too concentrated.
	The film could have been left in the developer for too long.
Fogged film	Light leakage in the darkroom, faulty safe lighting or poor film storage.
	Use of old film as a result of poor stock control.

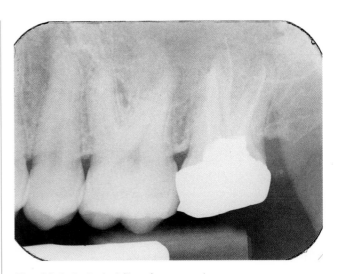

Fig. 19.2 Periapical film of upper molars.

■ *What is wrong with the film?*

The periapical film is too pale. There is insufficient contrast between enamel, dentine and bone and the background is not sufficiently black.

■ *How might this error have been caused?*

The film can be too pale for two reasons, each of which has a number of possible explanations:

Reason	Possible causes
Underexposure	Usually the time of the exposure is too short because the incorrect exposure setting has been selected or the timer switch has not been depressed throughout the exposure.
	The X-ray set timer may be faulty.
Underdevelopment	The developer solution could be too cold, too dilute or too old.
	The film could have been left in the developer for too short a time.

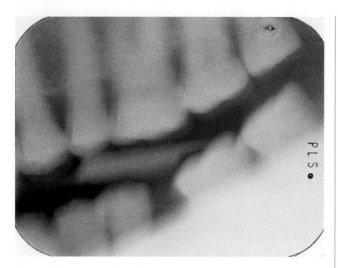

Fig. 19.3 Another bitewing film.

■ *What is wrong with the film?*

The bitewing image is blurred or unsharp and the molar teeth have been 'coned-off', that is, the corner of the film has not been exposed.

■ *How might these errors have been caused?*

Error	Possible causes
Blurring	Patient movement during the exposure.
'Coning-off'	The X-ray tubehead has been placed too high and was not aiming directly at the film packet. The straight edge of a rectangular collimator/spacer cone has prevented X-rays reaching part of the film.

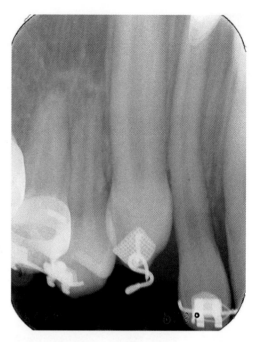

Fig. 19.4 Periapical film of upper canine.

■ *What is wrong with the film?*

The periapical image is geometrically distorted and has been elongated to such a degree that the apices of the lateral incisor and canine are not shown.

■ *How might this error have been caused?*

Error	Possible causes
Elongation	The film has been taken using the bisected angle technique and the X-ray tubehead has been positioned at too shallow an angle with respect to the teeth.
	The film could have been bent in the mouth by excessive pressure from the patient's finger supporting the film packet.

CASE

20 Ouch!

Summary

You sustain a needlestick injury. What should you do next?

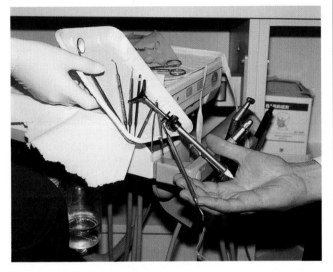

Fig. 20.1 An unfortunate reflex reaction.

Problem

You are writing up the notes after your last patient of the day. Out of the corner of your eye you see your nurse tip an instrument tray over the edge of the bracket table and instinctively lean over and put out your hand to catch it. The local anaesthetic syringe falls onto your hand. The needle sheath has not been replaced and the needle penetrates about 5 mm into your palm. When you pull out the needle the injury bleeds.

■ *What diseases of significance may be transmitted by needlestick injury?*

Most infectious diseases can be transferred by needlestick injury but the main concerns are hepatitis B, hepatitis C and HIV infection.

■ *What would you do immediately?*

- Encourage bleeding at the injury site and wash it with either 70% alcohol, antiseptic handwash or soap and water. Do not scrub the injury.

- Send the nurse or receptionist to ask the patient to return to the surgery as a matter of urgency.

■ *What is the most urgent priority and why?*

The most urgent priority is to assess whether there is a significant risk of transmission of HIV infection. Postexposure prophylaxis with antiretroviral drugs can significantly reduce the chance of transmission of HIV, but for maximum effectiveness it is recommended that it is administered within 1 hour.

■ *How could you obtain postexposure prophylaxis if required?*

Postexposure prophylaxis is only available following a formal risk assessment for each individual injury. This involves determining the severity of the injury and the risk that the patient is carrying HIV infection.

The procedure for obtaining a formal risk assessment varies with local circumstances. In hospitals, either the infection control consultant(s), hospital casualty or occupational health department will perform the risk assessment and provide the appropriate medication. Those in general practice must contact their local hospital casualty department who will follow their local guidelines. Each dental practitioner should know the contact number and name/position of the appropriate person.

When you phone you will be asked details of the injury and patient. You will then be told whether or not the injury is sufficient to carry a risk of transmission and whether a risk assessment of the patient is required. In general, a needlestick injury after a dental injection is sufficiently serious to warrant a formal risk assessment.

■ *What is the risk of developing HIV infection following a needlestick injury?*

On average the risk is approximately 0.3% if the needle has been used on an infected patient, but the exact risk varies.

■ *What factors affect the risk of transmission?*

The risk depends on the type of injury, the degree of contamination and the infectivity of the material transferred.

The risk of transmission is greatest with a penetrating injury. The risk rises if the needle has entered an artery or a vein because this allows a greater amount of blood to be transferred to the recipient. Dental local anaesthetic needles have a very fine bore and transmit very little fluid to the recipient of a needlestick injury, providing no pressure is being applied to the plunger. It is unusual for a needle to enter a blood vessel during local analgesia but because almost all dental syringes aspirate, potentially infectious blood or tissue fluid must be assumed to lie in the needle and local anaesthetic cartridge.

If the patient is HIV-positive, the main factor determining infectivity is the patient's HIV viral load, a measure of virus concentration in the blood. It is higher in late stage and symptomatic disease and reduces with effective treatment.

Splashes of infected blood carry a lower risk. Splashes onto mucous membranes including the eye carry a risk of transmission of 0.1% and onto broken or inflamed skin of less than 0.1%. Splashes of blood onto normal or healthy skin are almost without risk.

■ *The patient has returned to the waiting room with your nurse. What will you say and do?*

You should explain to the patient exactly what has happened and obtain informed consent to take their blood to screen for hepatitis B and C and for storage of serum. If infection is transmitted, it will be necessary to compare the patient's sample and your sample for Industrial Injury Benefit or insurance purposes.

Most patients will be happy to give a sample under these circumstances but, if not, you may need to point out your duties in respect to infection control and the need to protect your other patients. If a patient refuses to give blood, ask whether they would be prepared to let their medical practitioner take it. It is not unusual for patients to be upset, worried or angry about being tested for hepatitis. The general population have little knowledge of hepatitis but understand that it is a serious disease and may be aware that it is transmitted sexually. As a minumum, blood should be obtained to store the serum in case testing is required at a later date. As a last resort, permission to speak to the patient's medical practitioner should be obtained in case the patient has recently been tested for another reason.

The possibility that the patient might be HIV-positive will have to be addressed in order to assess the risk of transmission. This must be done in a sensitive manner, preferably in a quiet private room and with reassurance about the confidentiality of any answers given. The questions *should not* be asked by the recipient of the needlestick injury because it is difficult to be objective if you are anxious or distressed. However in a dental practice there may be no other suitable person to handle this issue and you may have to perform it yourself. As an alternative you could consider asking the patient to speak on the phone to the local casualty officer

responsible for postexposure prophylaxis, HIV clinic medical staff, an HIV counsellor, or other experienced person. Ask the patient whether they may be at risk of HIV infection. Use the information in the table below, and you may find it helpful to start by asking questions about nonsexual transmission first. However, questions may need to be asked about the patient's sexuality and lifestyle.

In practice asking these questions does not usually constitute a problem because in almost all cases there will be either no risk or a very low risk. Similarly, most HIV-positive individuals will disclose the information readily in this situation. If there is a risk, it is important that it is identified as quickly as possible in view of the need to provide prophylaxis within 1 hour.

■ *What are the risk factors for contracting HIV infection?*

The risk is attached to activity and behaviour, not to groups of individuals (see Table 20.1).

The exact risk must be determined in the light of local circumstances and the possibility of infection overseas. Africa accounts for 81% of all AIDS cases worldwide and the majority of individuals are infected through heterosexual intercourse. The highest incidence of AIDS in Europe is found in Spain followed by Portugal and Italy. Injecting drug use is a major cause of infection in these countries, while in the United Kingdom the major cause is men having sex with men. The risk of infection from blood transfusion is higher in countries which do not screen for HIV.

■ *If the patient discloses that they are HIV-positive, what information would you like to know from them? What is the significance of the answers?*

See Table 20.2.

The answers to these questions would be invaluable to the person making the risk assessment.

■ *If the patient indicates that they are not HIV-positive but may be at risk of infection, should you carry out an HIV test?*

Table 20.1 Risk factors for HIV infection

Type of risk	Risk activity	Relative risk
Parenteral infection	Transfusion	There is a small risk of infection to recipients of blood transfusion given between the middle 1970s and 1987. Most of those exposed will already have developed the infection and this is a very small risk for those who are not positive. Donor screening since 1987 has reduced this risk to a minimal level.
	Haemophilia	Recipients of Factor VIII-containing blood products before 1985 had a high risk of infection, almost 80%. Most of those exposed will already have developed the infection and there is a very small risk for those who are not positive. All UK Factor VIII sources are now screened.
	Injecting drug users	The risk depends on whether the needle is shared and how much blood contamination occurs.
	Needlestick injury	The risk is 0.3%, but depends on the type of injury, volume of blood transmitted and the infectivity of the blood.
Sexually transmitted infection	Anal intercourse	The highest-risk sexual activity. Condoms reduce risk but failure is common. The risk is greater for the receptive partner.
	Prostitution	Unprotected intercourse with a prostitute is a high-risk practice, but the risk varies greatly in different parts of the world.
	Vaginal intercourse	A risk to both partners but greater for the female. Properly lubricated condoms offer good protection
	Oral sex	Transmission has been documented but the risk is considered lower than for vaginal sex.

Table 20.2 Information from HIV-positive patients and its significance

Information	Significance
Whether the patient is generally well.	Patients with asymptomatic HIV infection have low viral load and lower infectivity.
Their CD4 (T-helper cell) count.	An indicator of immunosuppression, the stage of disease and effectiveness of treatment.
Their viral load and when it was last checked.	A direct measure of infectivity.
The names of any medications they are taking.	The same drugs would be avoided for postexposure prophylaxis if they are not being effective in the patient.
Whether their medication has changed recently and why.	Recent changes in medication may indicate their strain of HIV becoming drug-resistant and this must be taken into account in choosing the drugs for postexposure prophylaxis.
The address of the patient's HIV clinic.	To contact for further information. Obtain consent to do this and respect the patient's confidentiality.

No, definitely not. An HIV test cannot be performed without the patient's written consent and until after the patient has received appropriate counselling. This will not be achieved within the 1-hour time frame required for postexposure prophylaxis. However if the patient requests an HIV test or questioning reveals a significant risk, then on general health grounds it would be appropriate to refer them to a suitable facility for pre-test counselling as a matter of urgency. However, ensure that their blood is taken separately for the hepatitis screen.

■ *What is postexposure prophylaxis? Why not simply take the drugs regardless of the relative risk?*

The regimes for postexposure prophylaxis for HIV infection are complex and under constant assessment. At the time of writing a typical regime includes zidovudine (AZT), lamivudine (3TC) and indinavir, but this is likely to change as new drugs become available. Medication is currently continued for weeks.

The side-effects of these drugs include nausea and vomiting, headache, rash, tiredness and myalgia, insomnia and anaemia. These effects can be debilitating and therefore routine prophylaxis for every needlestick injury cannot be advocated.

■ *What if the patient indicates a risk of HIV infection to you but you cannot obtain a formal risk assessment within 1 hour?*

In this situation the first dose of the postexposure regime may be taken to allow further time to obtain a risk assessment. This would only be appropriate if there is a clear risk of transmission.

■ *What is the risk of transmission of hepatitis B by this needlestick injury?*

This should be minimal because all members of the dental team should be vaccinated against hepatitis B, and their antibody titre should be checked regularly and revaccination provided as necessary. However, if the recipient is not immune, the risk of transmission has been estimated at 30% if the patient is 'e' antigen-positive. Infection can follow transmission of as little as 0.1 μl of blood. Hepatitis B is so infectious that the degree of injury is almost immaterial.

If recent evidence of the effectiveness of the recipient's vaccination is not available, the recipient should have their antibody titre checked.

■ *Does this mean I have to give blood even if I know that my hepatitis B vaccination is successful?*

Yes. You must also ensure that your serum is stored, because you may need to show that infection was not present at the time of the injury.

■ *How can you determine whether the patient is infectious for hepatitis B?*

The blood taken from the patient should be screened for hepatitis B antigens and antibodies (Table 20.3) in order to assess the risk of transmission. The exact tests performed in the screen vary between hospitals.

Practitioners should seek the help of the virology or infectious diseases consultant at the hospital performing the test to interpret the results.

■ *What is the risk of contracting hepatitis C?*

The risk of contracting hepatitis C through a needlestick injury is 3% if the donor is infected. This risk is therefore higher than for HIV infection and the consequences can be severe. As many as 85% of individuals who become infected will become chronic carriers and of these, virtually all will develop chronic hepatitis. As many as 20% of patients go on to develop cirrhosis in the first decade or two of HCV infection.

■ *How can you determine whether the patient is infectious for hepatitis C?*

The routine test is for anti-hepatitis C antibody. Presence of antibody could indicate immunity rather than infectivity, but if the result is positive the individual has an 85% chance of being a carrier. If positive, infectivity is assumed and further tests are indicated. Detecting the virus in blood by polymerase chain reaction (PCR) can distinguish immunity from chronic infection but this is not a first-line test.

Table 20.3 Hepatitis B antigens and antibodies

Antigen or antibody	When found	Significance for infectivity
HBs (surface) antigen or 'Australia' antigen	Becomes detectable in late incubation and is present during the acute hepatitis. Declines over 3–6 months but persists in carriers, whether asymptomatic or with chronic active hepatitis.	Indicates infectivity though not necessarily a high infectivity.
Antibody to HBs surface antigen	Seen in recovery reflecting immunity against the virus. Also found in those immunized against hepatitis B.	Probably indicates no risk of infection. Denotes past exposure and immunity (including by active vaccination) to the virus and a *possible* need for further investigation to determine infectivity.
HBc (core) antigen	Only present in the liver, not used for determining infectivity.	
Antibody to HBc antigen	Found in acute disease, recovery and in carriers, whether asymptomatic or with chronic active hepatitis.	Indicates past infection but a high level indicates an infection risk.
HBe antigen	Becomes detectable in late incubation and is present during acute hepatitis. Persists in carriers with chronic active hepatitis but not usually in asymptomatic carriers.	Indicates acute infection or a carrier state of high infectivity.
Antibody to HBe antigen	Develops as Hbe disappears. Sometimes persists in chronic asymptomatic carriers.	Indicates either recovery from acute infection or a carrier state of low infectivity.

■ *Is prophylaxis against hepatitis C available?*

No active or passive immunization is possible at the time of writing and no postexposure drug regime appears effective.

■ *How may the risk of needlestick injury in the dental setting be minimized?*

Needlestick-type injuries do not always result from needles. Burs, broken plastic and hand instruments and other contaminated sharps all constitute a risk. You should:

- Ensure that all the dental team are trained in the disposal of sharps.
- Identify and dispose of needles and other sharps immediately after use.
- **Always** pass instruments with the sharp end pointing away from any person.
- Remove burs and ultrasonic tips from handpieces immediately after use.
- Pick up instruments individually.
- Never resheath a needle holding the sheath in a hand: use a one-handed technique or dispose of the needle immediately.
- Dispose of sharps into a solid container (approved to BS 7320).
- Ensure that sharps are disposed of by incineration and by an authorized person registered to collect such waste.
- Use heavy-duty gloves when cleaning instruments prior to autoclaving.
- Keep your working area well organized and uncluttered, with sharps in a separate area. Do not place waste material such as swabs or tissues over instruments. The bracket table shown in Figure 20.1 is not a shining example of good practice.

■ *What is your last duty before you can turn your back on this unfortunate episode?*

You must remember to fill in an incident report as required by law (The Reporting of Injuries, Diseases and Dangerous Occurrences Regulations 1986). Note the time of injury carefully. Evidence that procedures have been followed correctly would be important if a claim were to be made for Industrial Injury Benefit or insurance purposes in the event that you do contract an illness from the needlestick injury. Any incident in which acute ill health results from occupational exposure to isolated pathogens or infected material must be reported centrally.

■ *This injury could have been avoided if the needle had been resheathed. What are the advantages and disadvantages of resheathing needles?*

In general, needles should be disposed of immediately after use and this is the usual practice in most areas of medicine. When disposable syringes are used with needles they may be easily disposed of together.

In dentistry, resheathing a needle has the advantage that it may be reused for the same patient later in the appointment and at the same time is made 'safe' until disposal. If a needle is to be left ready for reuse it must be resheathed. Resheathing also reduces the risk of injury when removing the needle from the sterilizable syringe body, though it does not eliminate the risk completely.

Several methods exist for safely resheathing needles. In general simple methods are best and one-handed resheathing (picking up the sheath on the needle while holding the syringe in one hand) has this advantage. The sheath must still be pressed into place by hand to ensure that it does not fall off again. Holders can be used to support the needle sheath upright and these avoid both the need to seat it by hand and to chase the sheath around the bracket table with the needle. An example is shown in Figure 20.2. Alternative methods include proprietary devices where a sheath is an integral part of the needle or syringe. However, these still need to be used correctly if they are to be effective.

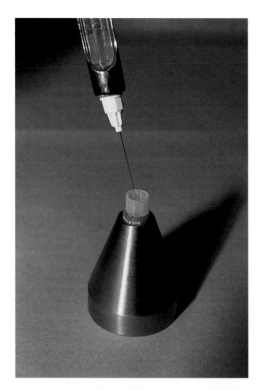

Fig. 20.2 A simple needle sheath holder. The holder is not intended to hold the syringe upright, only to hold the sheath during resheathing.

■ *This injury has ruined your day. This has all proved so complex that next time you might just wash the injury and ignore it. Why not?*

The main reason is the worry that you might contract HIV infection from an unsuspected carrier. The effectiveness of postexposure prophylaxis, reducing the risk of transmission by 70%, cannot be ignored. Also, it would be unethical for a dentist not to follow up the possibility of developing an infection which could jeopardize the wellbeing of his or her patients. There would also be a risk of transmission to the dentist's sexual partner(s).

A swollen face and pericoronitis

Summary

A 23-year-old woman presents in your hospital casualty department with a painful swelling of the right side of the face and neck. What is the cause and what treatment would you provide?

Further information on the diagnosis of soft tissue infection will be found in case 32.

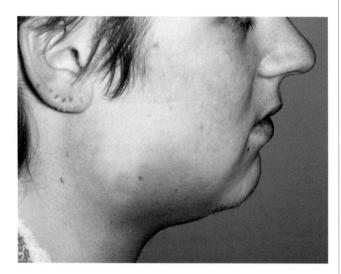

Fig. 21.1 The patient on presentation.

HISTORY

History of complaint

The patient has suffered worsening pain 'from her wisdom tooth' on the lower right side for 5 days. There has been some swelling of the gum around the tooth and she has been unable to bite together for a couple of days. Yesterday she noticed pain in the floor of her mouth and found that moving her tongue was painful. Today she awoke to find the facial swelling, she feels unwell and has difficulty eating, swallowing and opening her mouth.

She had an episode of pericoronitis a few months ago and is on her local hospital waiting list to have all third molars extracted. Until the swelling developed, she thought this was just another attack of pain from her wisdom teeth. She has not had facial swelling before and has come straight into hospital.

Medical history

The patient is otherwise fit and well.

EXAMINATION

Extraoral examination

There are palpable tender lymph nodes in the upper deep cervical chain and submandibular triangle. Opening is limited to 15 mm interincisal distance.

There is swelling below and around the lower border and angle of the mandible and extending back towards the neck. The swelling is hot, tender and very firm and a dusky red colour centrally. The swelling is not pointing to the skin. There is a marked halitosis.

Intraoral examination

Trismus hampers examination. The lower right third molar can be seen to be partially erupted, the operculum is swollen and pus exudes from below it on gentle probing. The second and third molars appear caries-free.

The floor of the mouth is very tender and firm on the right side.

■ *What additional examinations or investigations would you perform? Explain why.*

It is extremely important to take the patient's temperature to determine whether the infection is exerting systemic effects. She has a temperature of 37.8°C (normal temperature 36.8°C) and is, therefore, pyrexic.

There is a need to confirm that pericoronitis is the cause. It would be prudent to exclude the possibility that this is infection from a nonvital molar and tests of vitality should be performed. If there were a suggestion from the examination that a lower molar was nonvital, a radiograph might be indicated, otherwise radiographs would provide little useful information for diagnosis unless another lesion were present.

DIAGNOSIS

■ *What do these findings tell you?*

The combination of inflammation (swelling, pain, redness and heat) together with local lymphadenitis and pus seen intraorally indicate an infection. Pericoronitis is present and this appears to be the primary source of the infection. Trismus is an important sign, indicating that the infection or inflammation has spread to involve muscles of mastication.

The patient is pyrexic and feels unwell. These features indicate that the infection is exerting a systemic effect. Infection appears to be spreading relatively fast because the swelling has appeared overnight and there are already systemic signs.

■ *Which type of infection is this?*

It is difficult to tell because the tissues involved are deeply sited. Pus is draining from under the operculum indicating abscess formation, but this might extend into a soft tissue space or be limited to the tissues around the unerupted tooth. The rapid spread, firmness and tenderness of the tissues ('brawny' swelling) indicate cellulitis. This might continue to spread or develop into an abscess. There is probably a mixed infection with a local pericoronal abscess and a spreading cellulitis.

■ *To which tissue spaces may infection spread from a lower third molar? What are the boundaries of these spaces?*

Pus from lower third molars may track to many spaces and spread is unpredictable, depending on many factors including the angulation of the tooth, the size of the follicle, relationship to the second molar, degree of bone loss around both teeth and the anatomical relationships between the teeth, bone and muscle attachments in the region. Pus may drain into the mouth from under an operculum, into the buccal or lingual sulcus or into one or more tissue spaces. The routes of spread to tissue spaces are shown in Figure 21.2 and are described in Table 21.1.

■ *In what tissue spaces is the present infection tracking and why?*

This swelling appears to be in the submandibular space. The main infected tissue is not visible and lies around the submandibular gland deep to the body of the mandible. The swelling just spreads round the lower border of the mandible onto the face. Moderate trismus is typical. It is relatively common for this tissue space to be involved in pericoronitis.

There may well be early sublingual space involvement. Infection readily tracks between the submandibular and sublingual spaces around the submandibular gland and posterior edge of mylohyoid. In addition infection may spread

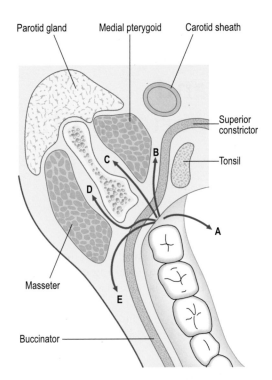

Fig. 21.2 Paths of spread of infection into tissue spaces from third molars: A, into the sublingual and submandibular space; B, into the parapharyngeal space; C, into the pterygomandibular space leading to the infratemporal fossa; D, into the submasseteric space; E, into the buccal space.

through mylohyoid which is thin, perforated by blood vessels and a poor barrier to spread of infection. There is not yet an established sublingual space infection because this would cause extensive floor of mouth swelling and deflect and limit movement of the tongue. Swelling from sublingual space infection would be readily visible in the lingual sulcus but causes considerable oedema in the loose tissues rather than the firmness and tenderness seen in this patient.

Table 21.1 Paths of spread of infection from lower third molars

Direction of spread	Tissue space	Boundaries
Medially above the attachment of mylohyoid	Sublingual space, A	Lies between the floor mouth and mylohyoid muscle with the body of the mandible laterally.
Medially below attachment of mylohyoid	Submandibular space, A	Lies between mylohyoid muscle and platysma, with the hyoid bone medially and the lower border of the mandible laterally. Contains the submandibular gland.
Posterior and medial to mandibular ramus, medial to lateral pterygoid muscle	Parapharyngeal space, B	Lies between superior constrictor muscle and the pterygoid muscles with the pterygoid plates.
Posterior and superior, between mandibular ramus and lateral pterygoid muscle	Infratemporal space via C which communicates with the cavernous sinus	Base of skull superiorly, laterally sigmoid notch of mandible and temporalis muscle, medially lateral and posterior wall maxilla.
Posterior and medial to mandibular ramus, lateral to lateral pterygoid muscle	Pterygomandibular space, C (and potentially on into the infratemporal space)	Lies between lateral and medial pterygoid muscles and the ascending ramus of mandible. Extends up to base of skull.
Posterior and lateral to mandible ramus	Submasseteric space, D	Lies between masseter muscle and the ascending ramus of the mandible.
Posterior and superiorly, lateral to buccinator	Buccal space, E	Between the buccinator muscle and skin

Pus from lower third molars tends to perforate the lingual plate because it is closer and thinner than the buccal plate. Infection is deflected to either the sublingual or submandibular space by the attachment of the mylohyoid muscle.

■ *Is this a potentially life-threatening infection?*

No, but it is serious. The patient's airway will be at risk if the infection continues to spread posteriorly. This would be potentially fatal and dyspnoea may develop unexpectedly and with great rapidity. Vigorous treatment of the infection must be commenced immediately.

■ *What is Ludwig's angina? Is this a risk?*

Ludwig's angina is a bilateral infection involving the submandibular and sublingual spaces. It is frequently caused by cellulitis when the classical 'brawny' (board-like induration) of the neck is seen. Spread of infection rapidly involves the epiglottis or parapharyngeal spaces and causes airway obstruction. Death may also result from septicaemia, disseminated intravascular coagulation or spread in the fascial planes of the neck to the mediastinum. Early diagnosis and prompt surgical intervention combined with definitive airway management are necessary to prevent serious morbidity or mortality.

■ *Is there a risk that the patient might develop this condition?*

It would be possible for this patient to progress to Ludwig's angina but this is not likely to be imminent and treatment will prevent this complication. However, she could also develop airway problems from spread via other routes.

TREATMENT

The principles of treatment of odontogenic soft tissue infection are described in case 32. It is necessary to drain pus, remove the cause of the infection if possible and provide antibiotics for selected cases.

■ *Where should this patient be treated?*

Admission to hospital will be necessary for this patient because she has systemic effects of infection and there is a risk that infection might impinge on the airway.

■ *Is pus present? If so, how will you drain it?*

It is unclear at this early stage of infection whether an accumulation of pus, as well as cellulitis, is present in the submandibular space. Incision may not be helpful. Infection at less important sites might be treated by vigorous antibiotic treatment and removal of the cause, followed by drainage, if required, 1–2 days later. However, because of the proximity of the airway, incision must be performed if there is suspicion of abscess formation. Even within a cellulitis there will be small collections of pus or necrotic tissue. Drainage is the safer option in this case.

The submandibular space must be drained through an extraoral incision, ideally 2 cm below the lower border of mandible (to avoid damage to the mandibular branch of the facial nerve). In practice this may not be the appropriate place and a soft spot centrally in the hard swelling is the best place to incise. Distortion of the soft tissues makes the position of the mandibular branch difficult to predict. Forceps or the incision must extend up medially to the mandible to drain the submandibular space. A drain will be required.

Drainage of the sublingual space is not indicated in this case and is rarely necessary. It could be achieved via an incision in the floor of the mouth (taking care to avoid damage to the lingual nerve).

Pus should be released from the pericoronal tissue by either an intraoral incision or extraction of the tooth.

■ *How will you remove the cause?*

A general anaesthetic will be required to drain the swelling. Fibreoptic-guided intubation may be necessary because of trismus and infection around the airway. In a more advanced case, with airway oedema or infection, intubation of a conscious patient may be required because paralysis for intubation prevents the patient from keeping their airway open voluntarily. Perforation of the pharynx during intubation is possible if it is oedematous or displaced and this might drain pus into the upper airway. Forcing the mouth open under anaesthetic may have the same effect.

It may well be possible to remove the third molar at the same time despite the poor access. This breaches the general surgical principle that surgery is best avoided in an infected field, but with effective antibiotic treatment postoperative complications are rare. Obviously the decision will depend on the difficulty of the extraction. Removal of the opposing third molar could also speed recovery and reduce the chances of another episode of pericoronitis. Removal of the lower third molar may have to await resolution of the infection.

■ *Would you provide antibiotics? If so, which?*

Yes, prescription of antibiotics is required for such a case. An initial bolus of intravenous penicillin and metronidazole would be appropriate with an oral regime for a few days afterwards. There is further discussion of antibiotics for odontogenic infections in case 32.

CASE
22 A sore mouth

Summary

A 55-year-old gentleman presents to you in general practice complaining of a sore mouth. You must make a diagnosis and institute treatment.

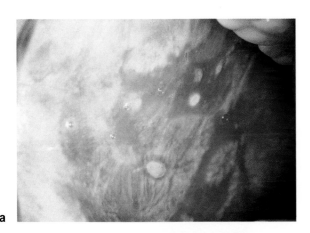

a

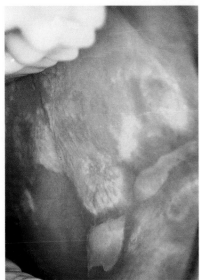

b

Fig. 22.1 a, b The patient's right and left buccal mucosa on presentation.

Complaint

He complains of an extremely sore mouth and the recent appearance of white patches on his cheeks. He thinks he may be allergic to his dentures.

History of complaint

The patient was fitted with a new set of complete dentures 3 weeks ago and since then his mouth has become progressively more sore. In recent days he has noticed the appearance of white patches on his cheeks. He had not noticed these before.

Medical history

One year ago the patient was diagnosed as a non-insulin-dependent diabetic and he has a history of peptic ulceration. Current medications are metformin and ranitidine. He is otherwise fit and well.

EXAMINATION

Extraoral examination

The patient appears fit and well. No cervical lymph nodes are palpable.

Intraoral examination

The patient is edentulous and his complete dentures are stable and retentive. The appearance of the right and left buccal mucosa is shown in Figure 22.1. Despite its abnormal appearance the mucosa is freely mobile with no evidence of tethering or scarring. Other parts of the oral mucosa appear healthy and the mouth is well lubricated by saliva.

■ *Describe what you see on the buccal mucosa.*

The buccal mucosa is affected bilaterally by poorly defined ulcerated red and white lesions. These extend from the commissural region to the retromolar area, as well as vertically into the upper and lower buccal sulci. The white areas are arranged as diffuse zones but some have reticular keratotic striae within them and around their borders. Irregularly shaped erythematous zones lie around the white areas and some have ulcers centrally. There are two large oval/linear ulcers approximately a centimetre in length on the left and one smaller ulcer on the right. The ulcers have yellow fibrinous sloughs on their surfaces and appear relatively superficial and flat rather than deep or punched out. No bleeding is evident.

■ *Suggest a differential diagnosis.*

1. Lichen planus
2. Lichenoid drug reaction
3. Lupus erythematosus.

■ *Justify this differential diagnosis.*

The combination of white, red and ulcerated areas alone is highly suggestive of one of these three conditions, though it could also be seen in a number of other mucosal diseases including vesiculobullous diseases. However, the presence of white striae as well is almost conclusive evidence that the patient is suffering from one of this group of lichen planus-like conditions. The lesions cannot be differentiated by their clinical appearance alone.

Lichen planus. From the clinical appearance alone, erosive lichen planus seems the most likely diagnosis. Lichen planus is a chronic condition, predominantly affects middle-aged or elderly patients and is the commonest of the three possible diagnoses. The appearances are typical of the atrophic ('erosive') form of the disease in which there are keratotic white areas with red atrophic zones and shallow ulceration. If this were lichen planus it would be slightly unusual. The lesions are usually less extensive and more prominent on the posterior buccal mucosa. Nevertheless, this could be a more severely affected individual.

Lichenoid drug reaction. Lichenoid drug reactions are side-effects of a number of drugs including the oral hypoglycaemic drug taken by the patient. Lichenoid reactions may be local (for instance in response to restorations) or systemic in which case they are usually caused by medication. Some features which point to a lichenoid drug reaction rather than lichen planus include a more severe reaction, extensive ulceration, asymmetrical distribution and severe involvement of the dorsum of the tongue. Lesions may also affect sites such as the floor of mouth which are less commonly affected by lichen planus. Lichenoid reactions may be clinically indistinguishable from lichen planus and the appearances of the buccal mucosa are consistent with a lichenoid reaction.

Lupus erythematosus. The mouth may be involved in discoid and systemic lupus erythematosus (SLE) and the oral manifestations of both types are indistinguishable. The clinical features resemble those of lichen planus and lichenoid reactions but some features may help in diagnosis. Lesions in lupus erythematosus often have a central ulcer or red atrophic area around which the striae tend to radiate rather than follow the random pattern of lichen planus. Lesions are also typically asymmetrical and affect the hard and soft palate and gingiva which are rarely involved by lichen planus or lichenoid reactions. Lupus erythematosus is much rarer than either of the other two possibilities and is unlikely as a new finding in a 55-year-old male.

■ *What further questions and examinations are appropriate? Explain why.*

See Table 22.1.

INVESTIGATIONS

■ *Is a biopsy indicated? Why?*

Yes. Ideally biopsy should be performed in all cases of lichen planus. In practice asymptomatic lesions composed of striae alone are often not sampled because they can be diagnosed clinically and no treatment is required. However, when there is extensive ulceration or atrophy or when the clinical diagnosis is less clear, other conditions need to be excluded by biopsy. When a lichenoid lesion is suspected but cannot be proved clinically, the biopsy may provide evidence to implicate a drug and this can be helpful when deciding whether or not to stop or adjust the dose of an important medication. Though not present in this case, lichen planus can form plaque-type lesions and these must be sampled to exclude dysplasia. Patients with high alcohol or tobacco consumption should have a biopsy to exclude dysplasia because lichen planus has a very low risk of malignant transformation. For this patient, an incisional biopsy is indicated.

■ *Which part of the lesion would you remove for biopsy?*

The centre of ulcers must be avoided because inflammation may mask histological features. However a sample of the ulcer margin may be useful and a piece including ulcer margin and red and white areas should be selected. Ideally some

Table 22.1 Further questions

Subject	Questions and reasons
About the medication	Date started, dose and any recent dose changes. Previous drug history for the last 5 years. Lichenoid reactions are sometimes dose-dependent and may be first noticed as a result of an increase in dosage. A close temporal relationship between starting a drug and developing lesions is good, though circumstantial, evidence of a causal link. Sometimes lichenoid reactions persist for years after the drug was administered.
About skin lesions	Are skin lesions present? Ask about and examine the flexor surface of the wrist and extensor surface of the shins. These are common sites for skin lesions of lichen planus and lichenoid reactions. The typical skin lesions are purplish polygonal papules with faint striae (Wickham's striae). They are usually very itchy. Severe lichenoid reactions may be accompanied by an extensive erythematous rash. Only a minority of cases with oral lichen planus or lichenoid reaction will have skin lesions on presentation. This is because the skin lesions often resolve spontaneously after a few years or with topical steroid treatment. In contrast, oral lesions may persist for many years and are often resistant to treatment. The skin lesions of lupus erythematosus are distinctive in distribution and appearance.
About the signs and symptoms of lupus erythematosus	Although this is an unlikely diagnosis the patient should be asked some questions to elicit evidence of lupus erythematosus. Questioning and examination should be more thorough if the oral lesions suggest lupus erythematosus by virtue of their appearance, distribution or the young age of the patient. Lupus erythematosus may be confined to the skin and/or oral mucosa (discoid lupus erythematosus). Lesions are well demarcated, round or oval red scaly plaques. The common sites are face, scalp and hands. There may be scarring and sometimes the typical 'butterfly' rash on the malar regions. Systemic lupus erythematosus has numerous signs and symptoms including those of discoid skin lesions (above), photosensitivity and hair loss. Internally there is vasculitis which can affect most organs. There may be glomerulonephritis, arthritis, anaemia and CNS involvement causing infarction or psychosis.

normal mucosa is always included in biopsy specimens, but in this case almost all the mucosa is affected. The specimen should be elliptical, about 1 cm long, 5–6 mm wide and an even 3–4 mm in depth. A biopsy specimen was removed from the left buccal mucosa and is shown later in Figure 22.3.

■ *What other investigations would you perform?*

Microbiological tests. When lichen planus or a lichenoid reaction become symptomatic or extensively ulcerated the possibility of additional candidal infection should be considered. The thick keratotic epithelium is more prone than normal epithelium to infection and in this case the patient is a non-insulin-dependent diabetic. A smear from the surface of the lesions on each side is an ideal investigation. Saliva sampling for candidal counts may also be helpful. This has the advantage that the organism is cultured for complete identification and sensitivity testing to antifungal agents. The disadvantage is that it does not specifically sample the lesion. In this case the patient is a complete denture wearer and is therefore more likely to have an increased salivary candida count. A smear is the better choice in this case and one was taken from the left buccal mucosa. It is shown in Figure 22.2.

Autoantibody screen. If lupus erythematosus is a possibility, an autoantibody screen may provide evidence to support the diagnosis. A serum sample should be sent for antinuclear antibody (ANA) determination. Four-fifths of patients with systemic disease are ANA-positive, often having high titres. A high titre of anti-double-stranded DNA (dsDNA) antibody is almost exclusive to SLE but is positive in only 50% of cases. In discoid lupus erythematosus this is less helpful in diagnosis because only a quarter of patients have antinuclear antibodies. Individuals with lichen planus or lichenoid reaction should have no antinuclear antibody. In this case the autoantibody screen was negative.

■ *The smear is shown in Figure 22.2. What do you see and how do you interpret the features?*

The smear is stained with periodic acid–Schiff (PAS), which stains the carbohydrate in fungal cell walls a magenta colour.

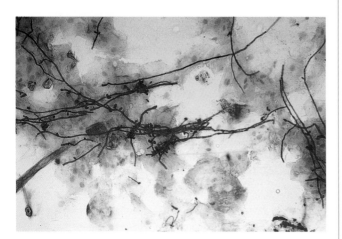

Fig. 22.2 Periodic acid–Schiff (PAS) stained smear from buccal mucosa.

(Gram stain may also be used to detect fungi; *Candida* stains strongly Gram-positive.) A sheet of pale pink-stained buccal epithelial cells is present, together with a few dispersed cells. Numerous dark pink branching fungal hyphae are growing in and around the epithelial cells. There are also several small round blastospores budding from the hyphae. The fungus is dimorphic and branching, and the size and appearance are typical of *Candida* sp. The patient has candidiasis.

■ *The biopsy is shown in Figure 22.3. What do you see?*

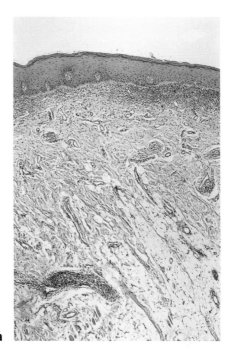

a

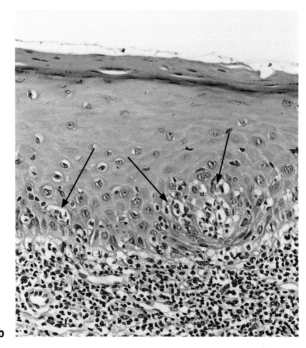

b

Fig. 22.3 Buccal biopsy; haematoxylin and eosin. **a** Low power view. **b** High power view.

The low power view shows mucosa with underlying fat. The surface epithelium is slightly thinner than normal buccal epithelium and has a surface layer of keratin. There is a well demarcated inflammatory infiltrate in a band immediately below the epithelium in the superficial connective tissue. The band is denser towards each side of the picture. (At this magnification the cells cannot be definitely identified as inflammatory cells but this is the most likely explanation for the very cellular zone.) There are also several foci of inflammatory cells in the deeper tissues, one particularly large one associated with a vessel near the bottom of the picture. The basement membrane is prominent.

The higher power view shows the interface between the epithelium and connective tissue. The very cellular layer can be seen to be composed of lymphocytes. Lymphocytes have infiltrated into the basal and suprabasal layers of the epithelium and caused the basal epithelial cells to undergo apoptosis. Apoptotic cells are visible as shrunken very pink cells with nuclear remnants (arrowed). There is no remaining clearly defined basal layer of small darkly stained cells and the cells lying at the basement membrane have the appearance of prickle cells. The surface is parakeratinized. Buccal epithelium is normally nonkeratinized, though a thinner layer than this may be present along the occlusal line as a result of friction.

■ *How do you interpret the histological findings?*

The dense band-like infiltrate of lymphocytes and lymphocytic infiltration of the basal cells with focal basal cell degeneration, apoptosis, loss of basal cells and a thickened basement membrane are typical of lichen planus. The deeper infiltrates of inflammatory cells around blood vessels suggests that this is the result of a systemic process rather than one localized to the epithelial–connective tissue interface. This suggests a lichenoid reaction rather than lichen planus as a cause. However, it is not usually possible to differentiate lichen planus and lichenoid reactions on histological grounds alone. For this reason the biopsy diagnosis is '*consistent* with a lichenoid reaction'. The dentist must ensure that this histological diagnosis is compatible with the clinical features and results of any other investigations before finalizing the diagnosis.

DIAGNOSIS

■ *What is your final diagnosis? Explain why.*

Lichenoid drug reaction with superimposed candidiasis. The clinical presentation is typical of a lichenoid reaction or a severe atrophic lichen planus, the diagnosis is supported by biopsy and the patient is taking a drug known to cause such reactions. The clinical appearance does not suggest lupus erythematosus and the autoantibody screen was negative.

■ *What drugs cause lichenoid reactions?*

A very large number of drugs may be associated with the development of a lichenoid reaction. Reactions to gold injection may be particularly severe and prolonged. Drugs of the following types cause lichenoid reactions:

- allopurinol
- captopril
- chloroquine antimalarials
- gold
- beta blockers
- methyldopa and related antihypertensives
- nonsteroidal anti-inflammatory drugs
- oral hypoglycaemic agents
- penicillamine
- some antidepressants
- occasionally other drugs.

■ *What treatment or advice would you recommend?*

Firstly the candidal infection must be treated. Denture hygiene must be checked and night wear ceased if appropriate. In view of the mucosal inflammation and ulceration, an antifungal agent should be prescribed and amphotericin or nystatin would be appropriate. Subsequently, intermittent chlorhexidine mouthwashes may help prevent repeated attacks of candidiasis.

Corticosteroid preparations would be helpful for the underlying lichenoid reaction. The mode of corticosteroid delivery is determined by the extent of the lesions, a mouthrinse being more appropriate than a spray or pellets when such a large area of mucosa is affected. The potency of the steroid must be matched to the signs and symptoms. These lesions are not suitable for treatment by the low potency steroids available to dental practitioners in the UK and either the patient's medical practitioner or a hospital unit will have to prescribe a more potent steroid such as betamethasone or beclomethasone. More potent or systemic steroids may be indicated if these prove ineffective. Continued follow up for candidal infection will be required because topical steroid use is a predisposing factor to infection.

■ *Would you change the patient's oral hypoglycaemic drug?*

Yes, if possible. First find out whether the causative drug can be withdrawn or reduced in dose. This must be undertaken by the patient's medical practitioner who will require details of the severity of the reaction and how distressing the patient finds the symptoms. As antifungal treatment may improve the symptoms, this discussion should take place after treatment and a period to assess the longer-term success. Unfortunately changing one medication for another of the same drug family may not prove effective. If the drug is changed it is important to realize that resolution may take place over a period of weeks or months and sometimes years.

■ *The patient complained of being allergic to his dentures. Is this a possible explanation?*

Such reactions are possible but statistically the likelihood is very low indeed. The oral mucosa does not generally exhibit contact sensitivity reactions. Two features suggest that this is not an allergic response. First the mucosa is usually evenly red and sometimes oedematous. Ulceration is possible but striae and keratosis are not features. Second, the palate and alveolar ridges in contact with the denture are not involved. In this case there is no reason to investigate the possibility further, but cutaneous patch tests with the constituents of denture acrylic, in particular methyl methacrylate are possible. Tests should be carried out in a specialist centre because these unpolymerized compounds are irritant and readily give false-positive results.

The patient had had a new denture fitted 3 weeks previously. One possibility which might be considered is that it has been inadequately polymerized and contains excess monomer. However, as in true hypersensitivity, the mucosa would be red and oedematous. Neither the signs nor investigations are consistent with this diagnosis.

CASE 23 A failed bridge

Summary

A 40-year-old man has a missing upper incisor replaced by a spring cantilever bridge. This has become decemented and you must assess options for replacement.

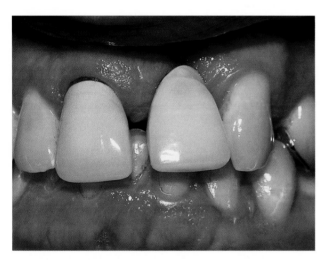

Fig. 23.1 The patient at presentation with the bridge which replaced the upper left central incisor reinserted.

HISTORY

Complaint

The patient complains that his anterior bridge has become detached. He would like it recemented or replaced.

History of complaint

The bridge had been satisfactory for many years but detached about 2 years ago. It was recemented and had been firm until yesterday when it fell off the teeth without warning.

Dental history

The upper left central incisor had been lost as a result of a bicycle accident when the patient was aged 16. It was completely avulsed and the adjacent upper right central incisor was fractured. The missing central incisor was initially replaced with a simple spoon denture and then a few years later by a spring cantilever bridge attached to full coverage crowns on the left first and second

premolars. The other upper central incisor was root treated and a post crown fitted. The present bridge is a replacement made about 8 years ago after the cantilever spring fractured. The patient has never had an upper left lateral incisor.

EXAMINATION

Intraoral examination

The dentition is in good condition with no caries and a small number of restorations. The upper left premolars are the abutment teeth and have relatively conservative crown preparations. There is superficial caries over much of the surface of the first premolar crown and a larger cavity at the distal gingival margin. The mesial surface of the second premolar is also slightly carious. Both abutment teeth are vital. The gingival condition is good except for bleeding on probing between the abutment premolars. Here the probing depth is 4 mm. The bridge can be replaced and the appearance with it fully seated is shown in Figure 23.1. The caries in the first premolar is exposed below the crown margin.

■ *What is the prognosis for this bridge? Why?*

Hopeless. Figure 23.1 shows that the cosmetic result is not good. The bridge pontic has moved buccally and upwards, probably a combined result of alveolar ridge resorption and distortion of the spring cantilever. It also appears to have moved distally increasing the median diastema. The abutment teeth will both require re-restoration and the first premolar appears to be very carious. In the long term, both abutment teeth are compromised by the risk of further caries and periodontitis.

■ *Why was this method of replacing the central incisor chosen originally?*

Although a well designed partial denture should not compromise the health of the remaining dentition, most patients prefer a fixed prosthesis without palatal coverage for a single tooth replacement.

The spring cantilever design was considered suitable for this case for the following reasons.

• It allows diastemas between adjacent crowns. Diastemas would have been present because the lateral incisor on that side was developmentally absent. A replacement crown which filled the available space would be too wide.
• The upper right central incisor was not a suitable abutment tooth for conventional fixed bridgework, having been traumatized, root-filled and post-crowned using a prefabricated post.

■ *What replacement restorations would you consider? Explain your choices.*

A new spring cantilever bridge. For the reasons noted above, the spring cantilever design remains a good choice and it has served this patient fairly well. However, the abutment teeth will require restoration and a further spring cantilever bridge may compromise the abutment teeth in the medium to long term.

An adhesive bridge could be supported on the upper left canine with the central incisor replaced by a cantilevered pontic. This would be possible because the lateral incisor is missing but would not normally be practical in this situation. This alternative has the advantage of minimal tooth preparation and allows maintenance of one diastema between the central incisors. However, success would be somewhat unpredictable, depending on the area of enamel available on the palatal aspect of the canine for bonding and the occlusal relationship. This might be considered the ideal medium-term or provisional restoration. It also has the advantage that the existing abutment teeth could be restored independently, reinstating their embrasures to help prevent further caries and periodontitis.

A single tooth implant would allow a restoration which was completely independent of the adjacent and abutment teeth. It would permit both mesial and distal diastemas and would therefore provide a cosmetically good restoration, comparable to the appearance achievable by a spring cantilever bridge. However, an implant would entail surgery, a more protracted treatment and much higher costs. A temporary restoration would be required until the completed coronal restoration was placed. One major advantage of the implant is that it should provide a successful long-term restoration. As with the adhesive bridge, the original abutment teeth would have a better long-term prognosis.

After discussing the options, the patient opted to replace the bridge with a single tooth implant.

■ *What are the components of a typical single tooth implant?*

1. The implant or fixture which is osseointegrated to the surrounding bone. Anterior single tooth implants are normally between 10 mm and 15 mm in length and approximately 4 mm in diameter.
2. An abutment which is attached to the implant by an abutment screw. Abutments are provided in various designs (according to use) and lengths. For single tooth restorations it is important to have an antirotational lock which prevents rotation between implant and abutment and crown.
3. The crown, which can be made of porcelain or porcelain bonded to metal. It is normally made on a prefabricated component which precisely fits the abutment. Typically, single tooth implant crowns are cemented to the abutment.

INVESTIGATIONS

■ *What further features require examination or investigation to assess suitability for an implant? How would you assess them and why need they be considered?*

See Table 23.1.

TREATMENT

■ *What precautions must be taken when inserting an implant?*

The implant is inserted into a hole which must be made with a drill matched to the implant. The surgical stent mentioned in Table 23.1 is used to ensure the correct angulation and depth so that the implant does not perforate the cortex. Careful sterile technique is essential and particular care must be taken to ensure that the bone is not damaged by overheating. Copious irrigation and slow drill speeds are required. The exact method of insertion and subsequent restoration depends on the type of implant and manufacturer. The implant must be left in place for 3–6 months to allow osseointegration before loading. A spoon denture would provide a satisfactory temporary replacement during this period.

Table 23.1 Features requiring investigation

Feature	Method	Reason
Edentulous ridge height and width, labial contour of ridge	Visual inspection and palpation	To ensure sufficient alveolar ridge remains for the final restoration to have an acceptable appearance. There must be gingival tissue where the gingival margin of the new restoration will lie.
Bone height and width Absence of bone abnormality at site	Plain radiography, ideally a periapical view taken using a paralleling technique and sectional tomographs to show bone width	To assess whether sufficient bone is present to accommodate the implant. A minimum height of 10 mm and width of 6 mm is required to place a standard 4 mm diameter implant. Tomographs and palpation detect concavities in the labial plate of bone resulting from resorptive remodelling of the ridge. These would dictate implant angulation because the implant must lie inside the cortical plates.
Desired result from functional and aesthetic point of view	Ideally, mock-up the final result as a provisional restoration or construct a diagnostic wax-up. Check the occlusion. Remember to check the old restoration and copy any desirable features	To assess the appearance of the final result and assess the relationship of the crown position to the implant position. Models are used to construct a surgical stent to facilitate ideal positioning of the implant.

■ *Figure 23.2 shows the result 3 years after completion and Figure 23.3 the corresponding radiograph. Is the implant osseointegrated and successful? How can you tell?*

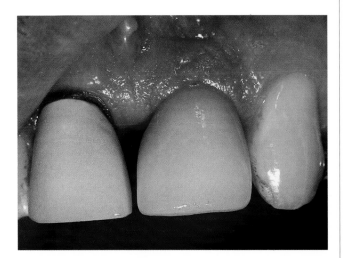

Fig. 23.2 The final result 3 years after completion.

Osseointegration is the direct structural and functional connection between living bone and the surface of a load-carrying implant. This implant was firm and symptomless and appears successful radiographically. There is bone in close apposition to the implant surface along its whole length. The end of the implant is level with, or only just above, the surrounding bone. Failure would be indicated by mobility, peri-implant radiolucency or progressive marginal bone loss.

■ *What factors are important in achieving and maintaining osseointegration and why?*

See Table 23.2.

■ *At each review, how would you determine whether the implant is successful?*

- The implant is immobile when tested clinically.
- A periapical radiograph does not reveal any peri-implant radiolucency.
- Radiographs taken at annual visits should reveal a steady crestal bone level after the first year of loading. This can only be assessed using periapical radiographs taken by the paralleling technique.
- Vertical bone loss, assessed radiographically, should be less than 0.2 mm annually in subsequent years
- Absence of signs and symptoms such as pain, infections, or, for mandibular implants, neuropathies, paraesthesia or a violation of the mandibular canal.
- The cosmetic result remains acceptable.

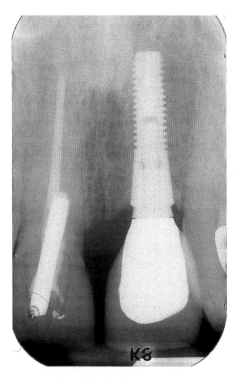

Fig. 23.3 Periapical radiograph taken 3 years after completion.

Table 23.2 Factors important in achieving and maintaining osseointegration

Factor	Reason
Implant biocompatibility and design	Implants of pure titanium osseointegrate successfully. Titanium alloys and hydroxyapatite are also used but may be less effective.
Implant surface characteristics	A degree of surface roughness is desirable for osseointegration and much research is currently directed at enhancing optimal surface characteristics. Currently used implant surfaces include machined, blasted, etched, plasma-sprayed or hydroxyapatite-coated types. It is unclear whether any of these offer a significant advantage.
Surgical technique	It is vital that the bone is not overheated during the preparation process. Elevation of the temperature to 47°C for a short period of time will cause bone cell death, subsequent bone resorption and failure of integration.
Bone quality	It is important that the implant is stable immediately after placement. Mobility induces fibrous tissue encapsulation rather than osseointegration.
Loading of the implant	It is generally recommended that the implant is not loaded for several months after placement, e.g. 3 months in the mandible and 6 months in the maxilla. However, this is dependent upon bone quality, implant dimensions and type of loading.
Occlusion	Overloading can induce loss of osseointegration or component failure.
Maintenance care	The patient must achieve and maintain a good level of oral hygiene to avoid peri-implant disease. Regular recall visits are recommended.

CASE
24 An adverse reaction

Summary

A 58-year-old lady feels very ill during routine dental treatment in your general dental practice. What would you do? What is the cause?

HISTORY

Complaint

The patient is to have a crown preparation performed on her lower second molar and a very small amalgam placed in an upper premolar on the same side. You have given an infiltration of 1.0 ml of lignocaine 2% with adrenaline 1:80 000 (12.5 μg/ml) and used a further 2-ml cartridge to give an inferior dental and lingual nerve block. Having finished injecting you turn away to prepare some instruments.

Almost immediately the patient says she feels ill. She is clearly apprehensive and is holding her chest complaining of palpitations.

Dental treatment history

The patient is in the middle of her first course of treatment for many years. She has been scared about visiting a dentist for some years. You have started a course of treatment and carried out several simple restorative procedures. You saw her only 2 days ago to insert several amalgams, using 3 cartridges of local anaesthetic. These restorations and one extraction have all been carried out under local anaesthesia using lignocaine 2% with adrenaline 1:80 000.

Medical history

The patient is apparently fit and well. The medical history records no allergies.

■ *What would you do?*

- Reassure the patient; encourage regular breathing.
- Lie her supine or slightly head down.
- Feel skin and take pulse.
- Prepare oxygen in case it is needed.

This applies unless the patient were pregnant or obese in which case lying flat on her side would be appropriate.

■ *One minute later the patient feels no improvement. What would you do?*

- Take blood pressure and monitor pulse.
- Check for pallor.
- Check for rash or urticaria.
- Wait and observe for dyspnoea while considering possible causes.

■ *What causes would you consider?*

The local anaesthetic appears to be the most likely cause of her symptoms because they started immediately after the inferior dental block. However, vasovagal attacks are very common and a medical problem unrelated to dentistry cannot be excluded. Thus, possible causes include:
- vasovagal attack
- adverse reaction to local anaesthetic
- hypersensitivity reaction
- myocardial infarct or anginal attack.

■ *Is this a vasovagal attack? Explain why?*

The features of a vasovagal attack are pallor, apprehension, restlessness, nausea, bradycardia, weak slow pulse and loss of consciousness (faint). The loss of consciousness may be immediate. In more severe attacks there may be clonic muscle contractions or rigidity as a result of cerebral hypoxia. None of these symptoms are seen in this patient. In addition, vasovagal attacks are usually caused by fear or anxiety and so may precede injection. Patients will usually be able to explain that they feel faint, either before or after the attack.

■ *Is this a myocardial infarct?*

No. The symptoms and signs of myocardial infarct are crushing central chest pain, sometimes radiating to arm or neck, dyspnoea and possibly vomiting which may be followed by cardiac arrest. There is usually, though not always, a history of angina, coronary artery disease or hypertension. Further information on cardiac arrest will be found in case 9.

■ *What are the unwanted effects of local anaesthesia with lignocaine and adrenaline? What are their causes and signs and symptoms?*

See Table 24.1.

While these possibilities run through your mind, the patient remains conscious but nervous and agitated. She gradually calms and says that the palpitations are reducing. She takes a few breaths of oxygen but refuses more after a few minutes and says that she feels better. Her pulse is 105 beats/min and her blood pressure is 140/90.

Table 24.1 Unwanted effects of local anaesthesia

Type of reaction	Unwanted effect	Signs and symptoms
Immediate	Neuralgic pain from needle penetrating nerve.	Electric shock pain on injection, sometimes followed by prolonged anaesthesia.
	Vasomotor effect of intravascular injection of vasoconstrictor.	Tachycardia without hypertension, in overdose arryhthmias. Occasionally, skin blanching on face or neck in the event of arterial injection.
	Facial paralysis from intraparotid injection.	Paralysis of one or more branches of facial nerve; may mimic Bell's palsy.
	Anaphylaxis due to hypersensitivity to anaesthetic solution.	Anaphylactic shock, local or systemic oedema, urticaria, asthma, hypotension, pulmonary oedema, tachycardia, breathlessness and circulatory collapse.
	Drug interaction.	Though theoretically many are possible none are practical possibilities at normal dosage.
	Central nervous system stimulation or depression caused by overdose of lignocaine.	Only seen in **large** overdose. Sometimes initial apprehension, excitability or confusion or muscle spasm followed by respiratory and cardiac depression.
	Rare complications such as needle breakage or infection.	
Delayed	Trismus or local trauma from injection, haematoma formation or damage to analgesic tissue caused by the patient.	Vary with effect.
	Transmission of infection.	Vary with infection.

DIFFERENTIAL DIAGNOSIS

■ *What is your differential diagnosis and why?*

Intravascular injection is the most likely diagnosis, the patient's symptoms being caused by the vasoconstrictor component of the local anaesthetic. The solution contains 1:80 000 adrenaline which causes tachycardia felt by the patient as palpitations. Intravascular injection is most common after inferior dental blocks and posterior superior dental blocks because of the high vascularity of the injection site.

Anxiety can itself produce a significant level of adrenaline but levels rise more slowly and the patient would have to be very nervous, positively phobic, to generate endogenous adrenaline to the levels found in intravascular injection of local anaesthetic. This patient is nervous but has recently accepted routine dental treatment without problems. A vasovagal attack would be a much more likely effect of marked anxiety.

■ *Could the local anaesthetic given 2 days ago contribute to this reaction?*

No, the adrenaline will have been rapidly removed into the circulation from the site of injection in spite of its intrinsic vasoconstrictor effect. Its action is then terminated quickly by reuptake into noradrenergic fibres and other cells and tissues. Metabolism takes place within these at various sites throughout the body by the action of the enzyme catechol-O-methyl transferase and to a much lesser degree by monoamine oxidase in the liver before undergoing renal excretion.

As far as the local anaesthetic component is concerned, the symptoms experienced by this patient are not typical of an overdose and, in any event, the half-life of lignocaine is only of the order of 90 minutes. We can therefore safely rule out any question of this event being related to either the local anaesthetic or vasoconstrictor given at the previous appointment.

■ *Is an overdose possible? What are the maximum recommended doses of local anaesthetic solutions used in dentistry?*

Although theoretically possible, it is actually quite difficult to administer an overdose of local anaesthetic in dentistry. The nature of the cartridge syringe and needle system used means that doses can be accurately counted and monitored and the need to change a cartridge affords 'thinking time' for the operator. This is in contrast to the other areas of the body where large volumes of drug can be administered into body spaces more easily.

However, we cannot be complacent. In recent years the recommendations for maximum safe doses of local anaesthetics in the head and neck area have been reviewed. Because of the vascularity of the region and recognition that vasoconstrictors do not hold the drug in place for as long as was previously thought, the recommendations have been rationalized and maximum recommended doses reduced.

It is important to realize that advice based on a recommended number of cartridges or fixed dose does not take into account different formulations. Some cartridges contain only 1.8 ml solution whilst others contain 2.2 ml and therefore 22% more drug. Thus 4 cartridges of the larger volume will contain almost the same dose of local anaesthetic and vasoconstrictor as 5 of the 1.8-ml cartridges. The concentration of drug also varies from preparation to preparation. Importantly, patients come in different shapes and sizes and fixed dose recommendations are based on the safety limit for the elusive 'fit 70-kg man'!

Current recommendations are expressed in the form of the maximum safe dose per body weight given over a period of treatment of 1 hour. Thus the maximum recommended doses are as shown in Table 24.2.

Table 24.2 Maximum recommended doses

Drug	Maximum dose	Maximum at any one time	Equivalent cartridges
Lignocaine and mepivicaine	**4.4 mg/kg**	300 mg	For 2% solutions about **eight** 1.8-ml cartridges or **six-and-a-half** 2.2-ml cartridges
			For 3% mepivicaine **five-and-a-half** 1.8-ml or **four-and-a-half** 2.2-ml cartridges
Prilocaine	**6 mg/kg**	400 mg	For 3% prilocaine about **seven** 1.8-ml or **six** 2.2-ml cartridges
			For 4% prilocaine about **five-and-a-half** 1.8-ml and **four-and-a-half** 2.2-ml cartridges

These limits apply to all preparations of local anaesthetic irrespective of the presence of or type of vasoconstrictor. It is no longer considered that larger doses can be given in one treatment session if the preparation contains vasoconstrictor.

■ *Immediately after calming down the patient claims that she must be allergic to the local anaesthetic. Is this possible?*

It is possible but is excessively rare. Only a handful of cases of genuine lignocaine hypersensitivity are recorded. A minority of older patients give a convincing history of local anaesthetic allergy, in some cases backed up by hospital investigations. This is because older preparations contained preservatives such as benzoates to which hypersensitivity was possible. The worst offending preservatives are no longer used, though very occasionally a reaction to sodium metabisulphite preservative is recorded. Patients can be tested for hypersensitivity to anaesthetic agents but this is only worthwhile when a typical allergic reaction is suspected.

Hypersensitivity is unlikely to follow repeated administration of lignocaine for dental anaesthesia. A much more potent cause is repeated application of lignocaine creams to the skin. Local anaesthetic pastes and solutions should be handled with care; the dentist is more at risk than the patient.

■ *Would a switch to prilocaine with felypressin in future be prudent?*

No, lignocaine with adrenaline has been used successfully in the past for this patient and there is no evidence of an idiosyncratic or allergic response to the preparation itself. Prilocaine produces a shorter period of analgesia and the patient should not suffer suboptimal pain relief because of the remote possibility of another intravascular injection. There is no evidence that prilocaine, with or without felypressin, is safer.

Such a switch would reinforce the patient's perception that she is allergic to local anaesthetic. A spurious history of allergy might compromise the patient's general health. Lignocaine is used in the emergency treatment of myocardial infarct and in many other medical situations.

■ *How can the risk of intravascular injection be minimized?*

Good injection technique is the key to reducing the risk of intravascular injection because it ensures that the minimum amount of anaesthetic solution is used. The solution should be injected slowly, reducing the risk of a bolus injection into a vessel. Using an aspirating technique is also helpful, and should be routine even though it does not always assure success; the narrow needle diameters used in dentistry aspirate relatively poorly.

It is impossible to completely avoid the tip of the needle entering a vessel. Indeed, in some very vascular areas penetration of a vessel is not the cause because the solution can be absorbed into the blood almost as rapidly as it can be injected. Nothing can guarantee the prevention of intravascular injection.

ANOTHER POSSIBILITY

■ *If the patient had had a genuine anaphylaxis, what causative agents would you consider?*

Anaphylaxis to other agents is considerably commoner than hypersensitivity to local anaesthetics. A number of other agents in the dental surgery should be suspected before the local anaesthetic.

Latex hypersensitivity is increasing in prevalence and is commoner in atopic patients and those who have come into contact with latex repeatedly, such as health care workers, those with spina bifida or those who are subjected to multiple surgical procedures. Rubber dam, gloves and even traces of rubber from local anaesthetic cartridges or drug vials can trigger reactions. Other less obvious items in the dental surgery which may contain latex are face masks with elastic components, amalgam carriers, plastic syringes, aspirator tubes, orthodontic elastics and emergency equipment such as ventilating bags and sphygmomanometer cuffs. These usually cause type 1 reactions such as urticaria, asthma or anaphylactic shock. Glove powder is a particularly potent method of disseminating latex allergen into the atmosphere and powdered gloves should be avoided to reduce the risk of allergy developing among the dental team.

In addition to latex, staff and more rarely patients, may develop hypersensitivity to acrylics, composite resins, dentine bonding agents, eugenol, cleaning and disinfection solutions and metal alloys. Almost all materials may be allergenic to some individuals. The worst offending agents usually have their formulations changed and the most notorious examples, particularly some synthetic impression materials and self-curing acrylics are no longer available in their original form. It is worth remembering that many of these agents are irritant as well as allergenic and skin rashes may not be true hypersensitivity reactions.

25 Fractured incisors

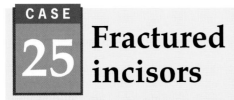

Summary

A 38-year-old man presents to you in your local hospital accident and emergency department. He has fractured his front teeth. You must manage the injury and outline a treatment plan for restoration.

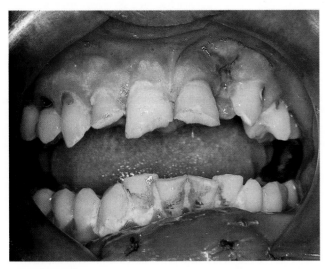

Fig. 25.1 The appearance of the anterior teeth on presentation.

HISTORY

Complaint

The patient's front teeth have been fractured and they are all loose. One tooth was knocked out and he feels pain when he bites.

History of complaint

The car accident occurred yesterday. The patient was sitting in the driver's seat when another car drove into his. He was stationary and not wearing a seat belt and was thrown forward, his lower face hitting the steering wheel. He did not lose consciousness and was taken to a local accident and emergency department where a laceration of his lower lip was sutured and no other injuries were found. At that time his teeth and jaws were not examined or radiographed and he has returned for a follow-up appointment with you.

Medical history

Prior to the accident the patient was fit and healthy, with only allergy to penicillins and erythromycin noted on his medical history questionnaire.

EXAMINATION

Extraoral examination

■ *How will you assess the possibility of a mandibular fracture?*

Fracture is suggested by:
- pain, swelling and tenderness at the fracture site
- bleeding, bruising or haematoma at fracture site
- displacement, step deformity
- change in occlusion
- mobility of fragments or of teeth
- difficulty opening the mouth or in lateral excursion
- paraesthesia or anaesthesia in the distribution of nerves involved in the fracture.

■ *How will you assess the possibility of a fracture of the zygomatic arch or facial skeleton?*

In addition to the features noted above, fracture at these sites may produce:
- facial asymmetry and flattening of facial contour (may be masked by swelling for a few days)
- step deformity along infraorbital margin
- anaesthesia or paraesthesia of cheek, nose, upper lip and teeth
- unilateral epistaxis
- subconjunctival haemorrhage with no definable posterior limit
- restricted eye movements and diplopia.

On extraoral examination you cannot identify a mandibular or facial fracture. The lower lip is swollen and lacerated to the left of the midline. There is no restriction or pain on opening, nor swelling associated with the temporomandibular joint.

Intraoral examination

■ *The anterior teeth are shown in Figure 25.1. What do you see?*

The swollen lower lip is just visible. The upper right lateral and both central incisors have been fractured. The upper left lateral incisor appears to be missing. The upper left canine is not fractured but has caries buccally and is mesially inclined. This inclination could predate the injury, in which case the lateral incisor may have been buccally positioned, or it could be a result of injury.

The oral hygiene is poor. This does not appear to be a result of injury because there are large accumulations of plaque, staining of the teeth, inflammation of the gingiva and caries buccally on teeth in the upper arch.

■ *What investigations would you ensure had been carried out at the patient's first attendance? Explain why.*

A posterior–anterior radiograph of the chest should have been taken to determine whether any of the lost tooth fragments were inhaled.

A soft tissue radiograph of the lower lip in the region of the laceration should have been taken before suturing. This would exclude the possibility that small tooth fragments have been embedded in the lip. Two views at right angles would be required to localize small fragments and surgical removal can be facilitated if radiopaque markers are taped to the skin before radiography. These markers may be used to localize the fragment at removal. Larger fragments of tooth in the lip are usually obvious on examination and debridement of the wound. Such fragments may cause infection or become embedded in scar tissue, sometimes deforming the lip.

Facial radiographs should have been taken to assess the possibility of an undisplaced facial fracture of the maxilla, zygoma or mandible. A suitable selection of films for this purpose would be a 10° and 30° occipitomental view, posterior–anterior jaws and a dental panoramic tomogram.

These films may have been overlooked at first examination if the fractured teeth were not recognized or if casualty staff concentrated on excluding more serious injuries. It is obviously undesirable for the patient to undergo radiography again.

You should ask the patient whether he has the lost tooth or any tooth fragments. These can be matched to the fractures to see whether other pieces are missing and to see whether a root fragment remains in the upper left lateral incisor socket.

■ *What features of the anterior teeth are important at examination? How would you examine them?*

Mobility of the teeth. The teeth should be tested for mobility in a buccopalatal direction, using a hard instrument, such as a mirror handle, and not the fingers which are too soft to detect small increases in movement. The degree of movement, if any, and the position of the fulcrum of movement should be noted. All upper and lower anterior teeth should be checked. In this case, all three fractured incisor teeth were mobile 1–2 mm, apparently about a fulcrum close to their apices. When the upper left central incisor was assessed for mobility, all three incisors moved together and caused pain.

The occlusion should be assessed to determine whether all teeth make contact in a stable intercuspal occlusion and that no pain is elicited on closing or in excursive movements. The patient noted no pain on closing into an intercuspal position, but in protrusion and lateral excursion he reported severe pain in the upper anterior region.

The degree of fracture of the teeth should be assessed by inspection. Though it is not visible in Figure 25.1, the pulps of all three fractured teeth were involved in the fracture line (class III fracture). The pulpal exposures were relatively large.

Percussion sounds of the teeth to detect any tenderness and to assess the sound. The percussion sounds of the

incisors were dull compared with the upper right canine and premolars, and that of the upper left canine was higher pitched. All upper and lower anterior teeth should be checked.

Test the vitality of the anterior teeth. As for mobility and percussion, all upper and lower anterior teeth should be checked. Following trauma there may be a period of apparent loss of vitality on testing with hot and cold stimuli or electric pulp tester (*concussion*). Nevertheless, the readings serve as a baseline against which subsequent tests may be compared. None of the incisors nor the upper left canine gave a positive response to ethyl chloride or electric pulp tester.

■ *How do you interpret these findings?*

The mobility of the incisors about a point close to their apex suggests luxation injury rather than root fracture, in which the fulcrum of movement is more coronally placed. This finding is consistent with the coronal fractures as, unless injury is severe, crown fracture is not usually accompanied by root fracture because the energy of the blow is absorbed by the crown. The fractured teeth have exposed pulps and their vitality is unlikely to affect treatment. The remaining teeth are probably concussed but this can only be diagnosed retrospectively as they start to respond to testing. The dull percussion sounds indicate a widened periodontal space, probably through oedema.

The mobility of the incisors as a group suggests an alveolar fracture. This is not displaced as the intercuspal position is painless and apparently normal. However, in lateral excursion and protrusion the patient felt pain as he occluded on the incisor crowns and moved the fragment. An alveolar fracture would also account for the dull percussion sounds (though periodontal ligament oedema could also cause it). The mesial inclination and high percussion sound of the left canine could indicate a lateral luxation injury or intrusion with impaction of the root in bone.

INVESTIGATIONS

■ *What investigations would you perform?*

Intraoral radiographs are required and should include an upper standard occlusal and periapical radiographs of all the upper and lower anterior teeth. The occlusal view and periapicals of the upper teeth are shown in Figure 25.2.

■ *What do the radiographs show?*

The occlusal radiograph shows that the upper left lateral incisor is fractured and intruded rather than avulsed. There is a curved alveolar fracture line running across the premaxilla, extending from the upper right to upper left lateral incisor. It is most obvious where it crosses the roots of the central incisors just above their apices. No root fractures are evident. The upper left canine has suffered a lateral luxation injury; the outline of the original socket can be seen most clearly on the mesial side of the apex. There is also caries distally in the canine.

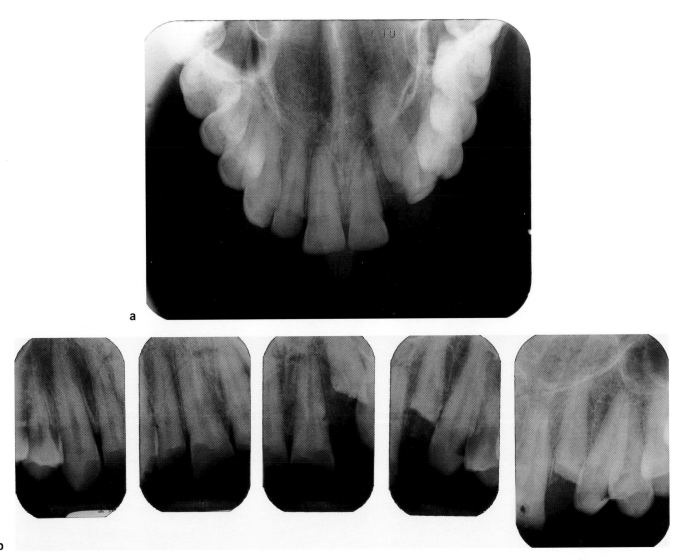

a

b

Fig. 25.2 **a** Upper standard occlusal, and **b** periapical radiographs of the upper incisors and canine teeth.

■ *What emergency treatment would you provide?*

The fractured alveolar process must be immobilized to alleviate pain and promote healing, and this is most easily achieved with an orthodontic wire and composite splint. The splint used in this case is shown in Figure 25.3. No displacement was present and so no reduction was required. The laterally luxated upper left canine requires repositioning before splinting either by manual manipulation or surgically. Manual manipulation was not possible and forceps were used to move the root past a bony obstruction and back into its correct position.

If it is accessible without disturbing the fracture, the upper left lateral incisor root should be surgically extracted as soon as possible.

The upper left canine has a closed apex and either the luxation injury itself or the surgical repositioning will almost certainly cause loss of pulp vitality. Therefore, the pulp must be extirpated from this tooth as soon as possible and a calcium hydroxide dressing placed. Calcium hydroxide has the potential to reduce the risk of root resorption. In addition the pulps must also be removed from the fractured incisors. These also have closed apices, the pulps have been exposed to infection for 24 hours and the exposures are large. In

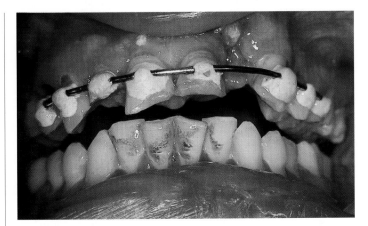

Fig. 25.3 Wire and composite splint in position.

addition, infection in the fracture line must be avoided. Again, the root canals can be dressed with calcium hydroxide paste and the teeth restored temporarily with composite, carefully checking the occlusion so as not to precipitate further trauma.

A chlorhexidine mouthwash should be prescribed for use until the tissues have healed sufficiently to allow oral hygiene procedures. There is no indication to prescribe antibiotics unless the lip wound was contaminated.

Table 25.1 Types of temporary replacement to be considered

Type of prosthesis	Advantages	Disadvantages
Partial acrylic denture of Every type	Minimal gingival coverage, easy to make and cheap. Does not interfere with orthograde root fillings of adjacent teeth. Acrylic flange masks bone defect following alveolar remodelling.	Patients dislike removable prostheses and they may be difficult for some patients to tolerate. Will require relining following alveolar remodelling.
Composite or denture tooth bonded to adjacent teeth with composite	Fixed replacement with no gingival coverage. No laboratory stage, simple chairside technique. Allows orthograde root filling of adjacent teeth.	Bond may fail because enamel has already been bonded for the etch-retained splint. Difficult to mask space formed beneath pontic following resorption.
Rochette-type adhesive bridge	Fixed replacement with no gingival coverage. Simple cantilever design possible, easily removed by dentist for permanent restoration.	Thickness of wing required may conflict with deep overbite causing occlusal trauma in already compromised teeth. Bond may fail because enamel has already been bonded for the etch-retained splint. Difficult to mask space formed beneath pontic following resorption. Orthograde root filling of abutment tooth not possible.
Adhesive bridge cemented with an adhesive cement e.g. Panavia 21	Fixed replacement with no gingival coverage. Simple cantilever design possible. Metal wing thinner than Rochette	Bond may fail because enamel has already been bonded for the etch-retained splint. Difficult to mask space formed beneath pontic following resorption. More difficult to remove, may require ultrasonics. Orthograde root filling of abutment tooth not possible.
Heat-cured acrylic conventional type bridge	Fixed replacement avoiding gingival margins of teeth other than the abutments. Greater range of designs possible including simple cantilever or fixed-fixed design. Best appearance and restores the coronal fractures of abutment tooth/teeth	Difficult to mask space formed beneath pontic following resorption but bridge is easier to remove and modify with composite and replace. Requires tooth preparation and commits patient to a permanent conventional bridge. More destructive than adhesive designs though teeth are already badly fractured. Slightly more difficult to isolate with rubber dam for orthograde root filling of abutment teeth; bridge might need to be removed for treatment.

■ *How long should the splint remain in place? What should be done in this period?*

The composite splint should remain in place for about 4 weeks. This splinting period should be adequate for both healing of the alveolar fracture and stabilization of the luxation injury. Some authorities suggest that lateral luxation injuries should be splinted for slightly longer. This can be achieved by selectively separating individual teeth from the splint with a bur. The canine should not be left unsplinted if there is mobility or pain. It is desirable to remove the teeth from splinting as soon as is practicable because it is difficult to isolate them with a rubber dam for root filling. Permanent endodontics must wait until the splint is removed. If still in place the upper left lateral incisor root may now be surgically extracted without disturbing the fracture and replaced with a prosthesis for 6 months to allow alveolar bone remodelling.

Throughout this period, oral hygiene instruction and dietary advice should be given. Success of treatment during this period will determine the long-term options for restoration.

■ *What types of temporary replacement would you consider for the upper lateral incisor? What are their advantages and disadvantages?*

See Table 25.1.

In this case a temporary fixed-fixed conventional bridge was chosen, and this is usually the restoration of choice when several teeth are badly fractured. The upper right central and lateral incisor were also crowned, primarily because of the better appearance although composite restorations would have been possible and might have

been preferred if the oral hygiene had not improved markedly. The appearance of the final restorations is shown in Figure 25.4.

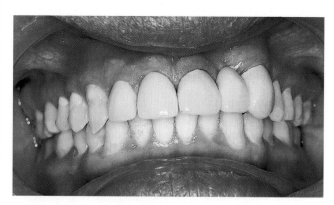

Fig. 25.4 The final restorations in place.

■ *What complications of the injury require follow up?*

In the short to medium term the other anterior teeth should be monitored for late loss of vitality. The main long-term problem is resorption, either of inflammatory type (following unsuccessful root treatment or persistent inflammation on lateral canals) or replacement resorption (without inflammation) which can lead to ankylosis. These processes start on the outer surfaces of root-filled teeth and must be excluded by occasional radiographs. The risk of resorption can be reduced by removing the splint as soon as possible to encourage early physiological tooth movement. Further features of resorption are covered in case 11.

CASE
26 An anxious patient

Summary

A 23-year-old student is referred to you for removal of her wisdom teeth. She is very anxious at the prospect of minor oral surgery and has been told that you specialize in treatment under general anaesthesia. Assess the treatment options and their suitability for this case.

HISTORY

Complaint

She has no complaint at present.

History of complaint

The patient has had several episodes of pain, swelling and bad taste related to both lower wisdom teeth during the last year. Her general dental practitioner has diagnosed pericoronitis and prescribed local treatments, but the episodes are increasing in frequency and severity and the last required systemic antibiotics.

Medical history

The patient has moderately well controlled epilepsy and suffered her last fit approximately 4 months ago. She is treated with phenytoin 300 mg daily. She also reports allergy to penicillin and septrin, both of which have caused rashes.

Dental history

The patient has had only a few restorations placed since the age of 10 years. Her general practitioner has provided intensive preventive treatment because she is so nervous. She can tolerate regular check-ups but has required no active treatment for many years. Her last amalgam restoration had to be abandoned on two occasions because of acute anxiety and fainting.

INVESTIGATION AND DIAGNOSIS

The patient has had episodes of pericoronitis and requires extraction of at least her lower third molars. Further details of the indications for removal of lower third molars and their radiographic and clinical assessment are found in case 16.

The patient has mesioangularly impacted but relatively superficial third molars and you assess them as being relatively easy surgical extractions which will require minor bone removal but not tooth sectioning.

ANXIETY MANAGEMENT

■ *What options are available for controlling patients' anxiety? What are their advantages and disadvantages?*

See Table 26.1.

Table 26.1 Methods of controlling anxiety

Method	Advantages and disadvantages
Behaviour modification	Simple to perform but time-consuming. Methods include identifying causes of anxiety (which may be visual, auditory or olfactory), modifying anxiety using desensitization techniques and a 'tell–show–do' approach. Works well in mild or moderate anxiety and for routine dental treatment but is unlikely to be appropriate for surgical extractions.
Hypnosis	Requires trained clinician and several relatively time-consuming episodes of training prior to surgery. Can produce pain relief as well as anxiety suppression. If patient has already received hypnotherapy their suggestibility will be known and the preliminary episodes may not be necessary. No after-effects and no drugs required.
Preoperative oral anxiolytic drug	Suitable for mild anxiety and restorative procedures but unlikely to be sufficient for surgical extraction. May be used in addition to other techniques if the patient is so anxious that they may not even attend for their appointment. Unpredictable effect in children.
Inhalational sedation	Can be combined with oral anxiolytic drug. Requires trained operator and team. Suitable for routine dental treatment in mild and moderate anxiety and especially useful in anxiety-related gagging reflex. Ineffective in nasal obstruction or if patient fears mask.
Intravenous sedation	Requires trained operator and team but relatively simple in comparison with general anaesthesia and easily administered in a general practice setting. Fast and with few medical contraindications or adverse effects. Patient remains conscious throughout procedure.
General anaesthesia	Never the method of choice for minor procedures because of the risk of fatality. Though very low, this risk is sufficient to contraindicate general anaesthesia for most dental treatment in normal individuals. GDC regulations require general anaesthesia to be performed in a specialized centre. May be required for patients with severe disabilities or more complex surgical procedures. Indications for general anaesthesia for removal of lower third molars are considered in case 16.

After discussing the options the patient elects to have her extractions performed under intravenous sedation.

■ *What constraints are placed on the use of general anaesthesia for dentistry?*

The General Dental Council made changes to its regulations for general anaesthesia in its *Guidance to Dentists on Professional and Personal Conduct* in November 1998. The regulations are subject to periodic review and failure to comply would render a dentist liable to a charge of serious misconduct. Though they affect directly only dentists registered with the UK General Dental Council, they outline sensible precautions for ensuring that general anaesthesia is only used as a last resort.

In summary, the guidance states that:

- The decision to use general anaesthesia should not be taken lightly.
- In assessing the needs of an individual patient, due regard should be given to all aspects of behaviour management and anxiety control before deciding to prescribe or proceed with treatment under general anaesthesia.
- The patient must receive a clear indication of the risks involved and the alternative methods of pain control available and provide written informed consent.
- Referral letters for general anaesthesia must provide a clear justification for its use with details of relevant medical and dental histories.
- A decision to carry out treatment under general anaesthesia must be agreed by patient, dentist and anaesthetist.
- Patients must be given clear and comprehensive pre- and postoperative instructions in writing.
- A written record of all procedures undertaken must be taken at the time and kept as part of the clinical record.
- The dentist must be assisted by an appropriately trained dental nurse.
- The dentist must ensure that the anaesthetic is administered by either a medically trained and registered anaesthetist, trainee anaesthetist or NHS career grade anaesthetist assisted by an appropriately trained individual(s) capable of monitoring the patient's condition and assisting in an emergency.
- The dentist must have a writen protocol agreed with the anaesthetist for the provision of advanced life support. The protocol must include arrangements for the immediate transfer of the patient to a critical care facility and must be agreed by that facility.
- Discharge of the patient must be performed by the anaesthetist who is responsible for recovery, either directly or indirectly through a properly trained individual.
- All involved in anaesthesia must train as a team for emergencies, and practice emergency procedures.

The choice of anaesthesia for extraction of third molars is discussed in case 16.

The patient had originally wanted to be completely unconscious for her dental treatment. Following discussion about the risks and alternative options, she decided to try sedation.

■ *Is epilepsy a contraindication to the use of sedation?*

No. Benzodiazepines (e.g. midazolam) are the drugs of choice and have anticonvulsant properties. In any case, this patient's epilepsy is well controlled. An epileptic fit under sedation is most unlikely.

■ *How would you assess the patient's fitness for intravenous sedation?*

The American Society of Anaesthesiologists (ASA) has a classification which is useful when assessing fitness for sedation or general anaesthesia:

ASA group	Definition
ASA I	Normal healthy patient
ASA II	Patient with mild systemic disease
ASA III	Patient with severe disease that is limiting but not incapacitating
ASA IV	Patient with incapacitating disease that is a constant threat to life
ASA V	Patient not expected to live more than 24 hours

■ *Which groups would normally be considered suitable for treatment in an outpatient setting?*

ASA groups I and II.

■ *Does this mean that ASA group III–IV patients should never be treated under sedation?*

No. Many ASA group III and IV patients may benefit from sedation because it reduces the patient's anxiety and, as a result, their endogenous catecholamine secretion. However, such patients should be treated in a hospital or specialist centre.

■ *What medical investigation would you perform?*

The systemic arterial blood pressure must be checked. 'Normal' blood pressure is 120/80 mmHg but small variations are common and the systolic blood pressure is often raised in anxious subjects. Hypertension which is well controlled is not a contraindication to sedation. However, patients with a diastolic blood pressure which is consistently above 110 mm Hg should be investigated before sedation is given.

When you take the patient's blood pressure it is 140/90, consistent with her anxious demeanour.

■ *Is this patient suitable for treatment under local anaesthetic with intravenous sedation?*

Intravenous sedation would appear to be an ideal adjunct to local anaesthetic. The patient has practically no experience of dental procedures, has a history of failed treatment under local anaesthetic alone and is anxious about the extractions. In addition, controlling the patient's anxiety by sedation will make the procedure easier for the dentist.

TREATMENT

■ *What is the drug of choice for intravenous sedation?*

Midazolam (Hypnovel) is a benzodiazepine well suited to dental sedation. It is soluble in water and presented in a 2-ml ampoule in a concentration of 5 mg/ml or in a 5-ml ampoule in a concentration of 2 mg/ml. Both presentations contain the same quantity of midazolam but the 5-ml (2-mg/ml) solution, being less concentrated, is easier to titrate.

■ *Are there any contraindications to the use of midazolam?*

Allergy to benzodiazepines is an absolute contraindication but is extremely rare. Some drugs interact with midazolam but careful administration of the sedative drug will minimize any difficulties. Drug abusers are notoriously difficult to sedate and treatment should only be carried out by very experienced practitioners.

■ *What is meant by titration of the dose? Suggest a suitable titration regime for a fit (ASA group I) adult patient being sedated with midazolam.*

Titration is administration of a drug in small quantities whilst observing the patient's response. Sedation is judged to be adequate when the patient looks relaxed, and displays a slight delay in response to questioning or commands (such as 'raise your arm'). There is often a degree of slurring of speech.

A suitable regime would be 2 mg of midazolam injected intravenously over a period of 30 seconds followed by a pause of 90 seconds during which the patient's response is observed. If sedation is inadequate further increments of 1 mg should be administered every 30 seconds until sedation is sufficient. Local anaesthetic can then be administered and treatment carried out in the normal way.

■ *What are the major undesirable side-effects of intravenous midazolam?*

Intravenous sedation with midazolam is an extremely safe procedure when the drug is administered according to the above guidelines. However, all drugs have side-effects and the major worry with midazolam sedation is respiratory depression. There is a dose-related decrease in both respiratory rate and tidal volume which is most pronounced in the first 10 minutes of sedation.

■ *How should a patient be protected from this potentially dangerous side-effect?*

Clinical monitoring by observing the patient must be carried out by both the dentist and a suitably trained and experienced dental nurse. The use of a pulse oximeter to monitor the arterial oxygen saturation and heart rate is mandatory for intravenous sedation.

All suitable pulse oximeters have 'alarm limits'. The minimum acceptable arterial oxygen saturation is 90%. If the alarm sounds the patient should be encouraged to take deep breaths. If this is not successful the airway must be opened (by tilting the head and lifting the chin) and the patient ventilated with the aid of a ventilator bag or mask. If breathing is still inadequate as judged by arterial oxygen saturation you should consider abandoning the dental procedure and administering the benzodiazepine antagonist flumazenil (Anexate).

■ *Why must a 'second appropriate person' such as a dental nurse always be present during sedation and recovery?*

To help monitor the patient's condition, assist with any emergency and act as a chaperon in case the patient experiences a benzodiazepine-induced sexual fantasy which might result in charges being brought against the dentist (or another member of the dental team).

■ *What postoperative care is required?*

At the end of the procedure, the patient is slowly returned to the upright position over a period of 3–5 minutes and helped to a supervised rest area. The patient must not be discharged until sufficiently recovered so as to be able to stand and walk without assistance.

The patient should be discharged into the care of an escort who must also be given written and verbal instructions.

■ *What instructions would you give this patient and their escort following treatment?*

- Do not travel alone: travel home with your escort, by car if possible.
- For the next 8 hours:
  — Do not drive or ride a bicycle
  — Do not operate machinery
  — Do not drink alcohol
  — Do not return to work or sign legal documents.

■ *Are benzodiazepine antagonists used routinely to hasten recovery after dental sedation?*

At present antagonists such as flumazenil are only recommended for emergency procedures such as countering benzodiazepine overdose and should not be used to hasten recovery. However, elective reversal of benzodiazepines may be helpful for some patients such as those who must travel some distance home on public transport. In such cases it is **imperative** that the usual postoperative instructions for intravenous sedation are given and adhered to.

PROGNOSIS

■ *Is the patient likely to require intravenous sedation for all future dental treatment?*

Not necessarily. Sedation will have ensured that the extractions were performed as pleasantly as possible and any existing dental phobia should not have been reinforced. The amnesic effect of benzodiazepines is likely to reduce the patient's memory of the whole procedure. During future visits for dental care anxiety-reducing methods should be used, so that eventually dental care can be provided routinely.

Summary

A 58-year-old lady patient of your general dental practice complains of a sore mouth with blisters. Identify the cause and outline appropriate management.

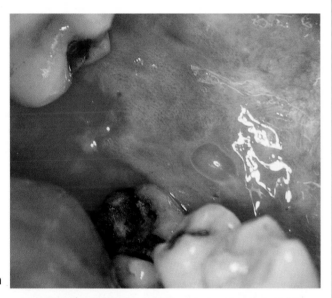

a

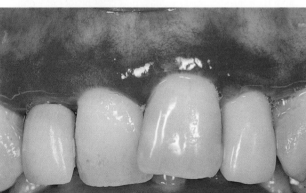

b

Fig. 27.1 a, b The patient on presentation.

HISTORY

Complaint

The patient complains of a very sore mouth. She describes blisters which last a few hours before bursting to release a clear fluid, or sometimes blood. The palate is particularly affected though lesions may develop

anywhere in the mouth and often follow minor trauma. Each blister heals very slowly and the area is painful until healing is complete. She often finds she cannot brush her teeth.

History of complaint

The symptoms started about 1 year ago and are worsening.

Medical history

She has had hypertension for many years and her elderly medical practitioner has been treating her with methyldopa.

EXAMINATION

Extraoral examination

A fit-looking woman with a blood pressure of 140/90 when sitting. Visible skin and nails appear normal.

Intraoral examination

■ *The appearance of the buccal mucosa and gingivae is presented in Figure 27.1. What do you see?*

The buccal mucosa has an extensive area of red atrophic mucosa posteriorly, possibly with small ulcers towards the anterior edge. The red area has an irregular margin. A small blister, a few millimetres across, lies near the centre of the buccal mucosa, just above the buccal cusp of the second premolar in the photograph.

The gingivae are also red but no blisters are present. The red area extends from the gingival margin across the mucogingival junction to involve the adjacent alveolar mucosa. The margin is poorly defined. The gingiva around all visible teeth are involved and the distribution of inflammation is not consistent with plaque accumulation as the cause.

DIFFERENTIAL DIAGNOSIS

■ *Which conditions cause oral blisters?*

- Mucous membrane pemphigoid
- Pemphigus vulgaris
- Lichen planus
- Erythema multiforme
- Angina bullosa haemorrhagica
- Epidermolysis bullosa
- Dermatitis herpetiformis
- Viral infections
- Trauma.

■ *What name is given to the gingival lesions?*

A band of red atrophic or eroded mucosa affecting the attached gingiva is known as *desquamative gingivitis*. Unlike plaque-induced inflammation it is a dusky red colour and extends beyond the marginal gingiva, often to the full width of the attached gingiva and sometimes onto the alveolar mucosa.

Some reserve the term for cases where the epithelium blisters or peels while others use it whenever the characteristic red appearance is present.

■ *What are the main causes of desquamative gingivitis?*

- Lichen planus
- Mucous membrane pemphigoid
- Pemphigus.

■ *Which of these conditions would you include in your initial differential diagnosis? Explain why.*

Either pemphigoid or pemphigus is the most likely diagnosis whenever there is a good history of blister formation. The most frequent cause of oral blisters is mucous membrane ('cicatricial') pemphigoid. This typically affects middle-aged and elderly women causing relatively long-lived vesicles and bullae (bullae are blisters greater than 10 mm in diameter) in areas of friction. Pemphigus vulgaris is less common and predominantly affects women in early middle age. In pemphigus it is unusual to notice long-lived vesicles or bullae, because the loss of keratinocyte adhesion which causes the disease makes the blister roof extremely fragile. Both diseases cause desquamative gingivitis. In this case, the history is more suggestive of pemphigoid than pemphigus. However, pemphigus must be specifically excluded by investigation because it can progress to extensive skin lesions and be difficult to treat.

These conditions would also need to be considered whenever a patient presents with chronic ulceration or erosion of the oral mucosa. This is because the vesicles and bullae often break down so rapidly that patients may be unaware of the blistering phase. Ragged tags of epithelium around ulcer margins would suggest that the ulcer was derived from a preexisting bulla.

Lichen planus is the commonest condition in the differential diagnosis and also affects the middle-aged. However, it rarely produces well-defined blisters and when it does they are usually on the gingivae. Some refer to this situation as *bullous lichen planus*. However, this is not a specific form of lichen planus. Bulla formation merely reflects separation of the epithelium as a result of inflammatory destruction of its basal cells by the underlying disease process. In this case lichen planus seems an unlikely cause. Blisters are a prominent feature and no white striae are present on the buccal mucosa or the affected gingivae.

■ *What diagnoses have you excluded? Explain why.*

Erythema multiforme is an unlikely possibility. Although erythema multiforme does cause blistering it is distinctive clinically. The pattern of recurrent episodes of acute blistering and ulceration, particularly affecting the anterior mouth and lips of young males, is characteristic. Occasionally patients, including the middle-aged, have a more chronic form of erythema multiforme and the diagnosis might be considered when other more common blistering conditions have been

excluded. Erythema multiforme does not cause typical desquamative gingivitis.

Angina bullosa haemorrhagica is the name given to recurrent oral blood blisters. The blisters usually affect the palate and are often long lived to the extent that patients burst them for symptomatic relief. The condition is diagnosed on the basis of exclusion of other conditions and the typical presentation, particularly the constant presence of blood as the blister fluid. In this case blood was present in only a minority of the lesions and the sites involved would not be typical. Angina bullosa haemorrhagica does not cause desquamative gingivitis.

Drug reactions may occasionally lead to pemphigus and pemphigoid-like presentations, lichenoid reactions and erythema multiforme. This patient is taking methyldopa which is commonly implicated in lichenoid reactions but these are lichen planus-like rather than vesiculobullous. Of these conditions, only a lichenoid reaction might cause desquamative gingivitis.

A number of less common vesiculobullous conditions may affect the mouth, but can be effectively excluded at this stage. Dermatitis herpetiformis may be associated with coeliac disease and is usually accompanied by skin lesions and usually affects the soft palate. The various forms of epidermolysis bullosa are inherited and most are accompanied by skin lesions from a young age. Unlike the skin, direct trauma is almost never a cause of oral vesicles or bullae. Viral conditions cause acute single attacks of vesicles rather than bullae and are usually accompanied by systemic signs of infection.

■ *What additional questions would you ask in the history? Why?*

Do you have any blisters on your skin? This is the most important question. Skin lesions, or a clear history of them, would confirm the presence of a systemic disease, may aid diagnosis and provide further lesions for investigation. Approximately half of pemphigus patients have oral lesions alone during the first year but develop skin lesions later. Lichen planus may be accompanied by a rash on the wrists, shins or back. Though the rash may resolve long before the oral lesions, it should be specifically sought in the history if lichen planus is a possibility. Erythema multiforme may be accompanied by the typical target lesions, though these usually signify typical severe oral erythema multiforme (Stevens–Johnson syndrome) which is unlike this patient's presentation. A history of onset following specific triggers (e.g. cold sore) would also suggest erythema multiforme.

Do you have any lesions anywhere else? Mucous membrane pemphigoid may be accompanied by ocular and vaginal lesions, the former leading to scarring and, if untreated, sometimes blindness. Eye and vaginal symptoms should be sought by questioning and, if appropriate, by examination.

If you were able to examine the patient you would find that she has no skin lesions and gives no history of a rash.

Table 27.1 Tests and special procedures

Test	Significance/special procedures
Nikolsky's sign	Some clinicians attempt to elicit Nikolsky's sign, in which gentle lateral pressure on apparently unaffected mucosa or skin (*not* rubbing the surface) raises a bulla. This is positive in vesiculobullous diseases but is somewhat unpredictable. In pemphigus the epithelium tends to disintegrate rather than form a bulla. If no lesions are present on examination it may be a useful way of demonstrating reduced epithelial adhesion, but it is often not necessary for diagnosis. Unsurprisingly, it is also unpopular with patients who are left with a large new ulcer which may take weeks to heal.
Biopsy	An incisional biopsy is indicated and it will almost certainly need to be investigated by immunofluorescence to differentiate the autoimmune blistering conditions. An incisional specimen removed from a vesicle or bulla margin or from apparently normal perilesional mucosa is best. Skin may also be sampled if involved. The biopsy must include epithelium and may be difficult to perform because the mucosa may disintegrate on slight trauma. The specimen should be either taken fresh to the laboratory immediately, frozen in liquid nitrogen at the chairside or placed in a special medium. Tissue fixed in formalin is useless for immunofluorescence.
Serum autoantibody determination	A sample of clotted blood should also be sent for indirect immunofluorescence to detect circulating pemphigus or pemphigoid autoantibody.

INVESTIGATIONS

■ *What special tests would you perform and what is their significance? Are any special procedures required?*

See Table 27.1.

■ *The biopsy specimen is shown in Figure 27.2. What do you see?*

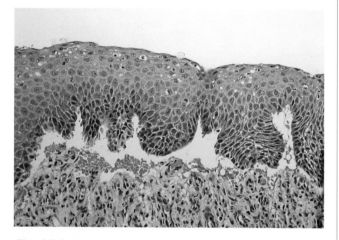

Fig. 27.2 Histological appearances of the biopsy specimen stained with haematoxylin and eosin.

The epithelium has separated cleanly from the underlying connective tissue in the plane of the basement membrane. A few erythrocytes lie in the cleft between the two. No cause for the separation is evident. The epithelium appears almost normal and there are only a few inflammatory cells in the lamina propria.

■ *The immunofluorescence stain for complement C3 is shown in Figure 27.3. What do you see?*

The immunofluorescence staining has been carried out on a separate part of the specimen in which there is no epithelial separation. A bright line of fluorescence runs along the basement membrane, outlining the rete processes of the

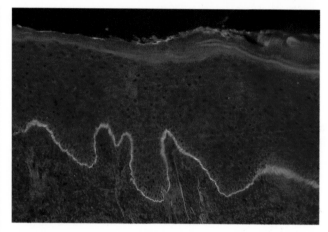

Fig. 27.3 The biopsy specimen after immunofluorescence staining for complement component C3.

epithelium. Immunofluorescence for IgG gave an identical result.

■ *How do you interpret these histological features?*

Separation of the full thickness of the epithelium at the level of the basement membrane, without epithelial damage, almost certainly signifies pemphigoid. Pemphigus is excluded by the lack of acantholysis and the level of separation. Lichen planus is excluded by the lack of basal cell degeneration and lymphocytic infiltration of the epithelium. The direct immunofluorescence indicates binding of immunoglobulin IgG at the basement membrane and activation of complement. This indicates pemphigoid in which IgG autoantibody binds and fixes complement. Taken together, these features indicate pemphigoid.

DIAGNOSIS

The patient has pemphigoid. There are different variants of pemphigoid but, as there is no skin involvement, mucous membrane pemphigoid is almost certainly the diagnosis. Bullous pemphigoid, linear IgA disease and epidermolysis bullosa acquisita are pemphigoid variants which very rarely affect the mouth.

TREATMENT

■ *How should this patient be managed?*

The patient should preferably be treated in a hospital environment, at least initially. This will probably be necessary in order to perform the immunofluorescence tests. Treatment of pemphigoid requires more potent steroids than are usually considered appropriate in a general dental practice setting. However, there is no reason why routine dental treatment should be transferred to hospital.

The patient should be referred to an ophthalmologist to identify and manage any ocular lesions which may be present.

Oral lesions should be treated with steroids. Occasionally topical treatment alone will induce remission using relatively potent steroids such as betamethasone 0.5 mg q.d.s. as a mouthwash. Patients must be warned not to swallow topical steroid doses and should be regularly checked for adverse effects. If severe, a course of systemic steroids may bring the condition under control to the degree that topical steroids are sufficient for maintenance.

All patients using systemic or topical steroids are predisposed to oral candidal infection and this should be monitored at subsequent visits.

CASE
28
Bridge design

Summary

A 28-year-old woman presents to you in your general dental practice with an edentulous premolar space on the upper left. She would like this space filled. What are the options?

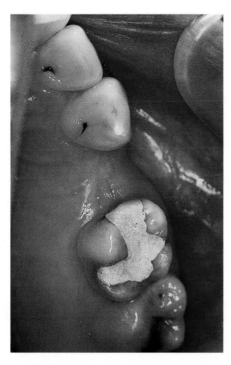

Fig. 28.1 The premolar space on presentation.

HISTORY

Complaint

Her complaint is the appearance of the gap. She would like it filled in time for her wedding in a few months time and requests a bridge.

History of complaint

The patient had all four first premolars extracted for orthodontic treatment in her early teens. After treatment with fixed appliances the premolar space was closed and the result had been stable. However, she then lost the upper left second premolar because of a combination of caries and root fracture following root canal treatment. This was about 2 years ago and she has had no replacement since.

Dental history

The patient first came to your practice 18 months ago, shortly after having had the second premolar extracted. You have made her dentally fit and instituted preventive treatment which appears to have been successful. No caries is present in any teeth and the gingival condition is good. The patient consumes a low sugar diet and has good oral hygiene.

Medical history

The patient is fit and well with no medical problems.

EXAMINATION

Extraoral examination

No abnormalities are present on extraoral examination. The premolar space is visible during speech.

Intraoral examination

The patient has an almost complete and well restored dentition with small or medium amalgam restorations. Although two premolars are missing, the gap is only a single premolar-sized unit of space because of the orthodontic treatment. This is her only missing tooth.

There is a mesioocclusal restoration in the upper left first molar tooth. The first molar and the incisor teeth are in class I occlusion, with canine guidance in left lateral excursion. The orthodontic treatment has left the canine and molar vertically aligned and there has been no significant mesial drift of the first molar in the 2 years since extraction. The features are shown in Figure 28.1.

■ *What alternatives are there for replacing the missing tooth and what are their relative advantages and disadvantages?*

The options are shown in Table 28.1.

■ *What specific features of importance with regard to restoration would you examine? Explain why.*

The degree of bone loss of the edentulous alveolar ridge is important. If this is extensively resorbed, an elongated pontic would be necessary to hide the bone loss. This might well be unacceptable if the pontic is easily seen during talking or smiling. This problem can be overcome with ridge augmentation prior to placement of the bridge, but this would prolong the treatment and make it considerably more complex. A diagnostic wax-up may help the patient visualize the potential result if resorption is a problem or the appearance is critical.

Size of existing restorations in potential abutment tooth. This is the most important consideration for minimal preparation bridges which require either no restorations or only small restorations in abutment teeth. Extensively restored teeth leave little natural tooth tissue to supply retention for conventional bridges. The quality of existing restorations must be known if they are to be used to prepare a core.

Table 28.1 Replacement options

Replacement	Advantages	Disadvantages
Removable partial denture	Removable for cleaning; cheaper than a fixed replacement; flange useful to improve appearance if significant bone loss has developed buccally; appearance can be good.	Patients rarely prefer a removable prosthesis and dislike palatal coverage. If poorly cleaned it will compromise the gingival margin around several teeth. Retention may deteriorate with time.
Minimal preparation bridge	Appearance can be excellent. No coverage of the palate required. Conservative of tooth tissue. Subsequent preparation for a conventional bridge is possible.	More expensive, significant laboratory fees. Not suitable if there is significant loss of alveolar ridge after the extraction. Must be cleaned in place. Average lifespan of restoration only about 5 years.
Conventional bridge	As for the minimal preparation bridge. Additionally, crowning adjacent teeth allows their appearance to be improved if heavily restored. Reasonable longevity approaching 10 years.	As for the minimal preparation bridge. Additionally destructive of tooth tissue.
Implant retained crown	Conservative of tooth tissue; no abutment preparation needed. Long-term survival rates are good.	Expensive. Involves surgical procedures as well as laboratory fees. Not an immediate result; may take 6–9 months to complete. Patient may require temporary prosthesis while implant integrates. Good quality bone and sufficient alveolar width and height required.

Inclination of the potential abutment teeth. A degree of vertical alignment is necessary to eliminate undercuts and allow the bridge to be made in the laboratory. Provided the teeth are fairly parallel this can be provided by preparation. If the teeth are not parallel, a fixed movable design is useful because it allows the restoration on each tooth to have a different path of withdrawal.

Reduced length of clinical crown on either potential abutment tooth. Tooth wear or repeated restoration may reduce the length of the clinical crown. There may be insufficient crown length to guarantee a retentive preparation. In extreme cases additional retention such as a post may need to be considered. However, post crowns do not make very good bridge retainers. They fail relatively frequently and should be avoided wherever possible.

Increased length of clinical crown on either potential abutment tooth. Recession makes crown preparation more difficult because it is difficult to prevent undercuts in long preparations. It may be necessary to place the crown margin some distance from the gingival margin and this might compromise the appearance if the margin were visible.

The width of the alveolar ridge is also important if implants are to be considered. For standard implants a minimum of 7 mm mesiodistal space between the adjacent teeth and 7 mm interocclusal space is needed. Particular attention should be made to the buccal contour of the edentulous ridge as a concavity would make implant placement difficult.

■ *What special investigations would you carry out? Explain why.*

Tests of vitality of the potential abutment teeth, in this case the upper left first molar and canine.

If teeth are nonvital, any bridge design would need to take this into account. If required, endodontic treatment would have to be performed before bridge construction. The bridge should not be made until root filling is proved successful. Also, it

would be a pity to have to weaken the bridge by making access to the root canals after placement.

Periapical radiographs of the potential abutment teeth are required. These are to exclude unsuspected caries, periodontal bone loss and other pathological lesions. They may also be required to assess the quality of preexisting root fillings or for root treatment if either tooth proves to be nonvital.

Study models are useful in some cases. They can be used to make a diagnostic wax-up to show the patient the likely shape of the proposed bridges and to mould a former to make a provisional restoration. They also allow the clinician to plan treatment, including abutment preparation and pontic size outside the mouth. Articulated models mounted using a facebow could be used to analyse the occlusion.

DIAGNOSIS

■ *What type of replacement appears ideal?*

The patient has indicated a preference for a fixed prosthesis and there seems no clinical reason to suggest any other option. A minimal preparation bridge is the most conservative option. A conventional bridge in this region would mean considerable destruction of the unrestored abutment teeth. Minimal preparation bridges carry the risk of failure sooner than conventional bridges, but a lifespan of about 5 years can be expected and a conventional bridge or implants could be considered then. There would be no advantage in providing a metal-based partial denture. The costs would be similar to those of a bridge.

The possibility of leaving the gap unfilled should also be considered. The adjacent teeth might drift into the gap or the opposing teeth might overerupt. These changes could be kept under review using study casts. However, even if the teeth did move, a prosthesis remains only advisable and not essential. This is a decision based on appearance and the final decision must rest with the patient.

What factors might make you suggest a removable prosthesis instead?

The cost is probably the most common reason for choosing a denture rather than a bridge. However a number of specific reasons might favour the removable prosthesis:

- Missing teeth requiring replacement on both sides of the arch.
- Mobility or significant periodontal bone loss or inflammation around either abutment tooth.
- If the patient is likely to lose further teeth in the short term, replacements would be more easily added to a partial denture.
- A high smile line with marked resorption of the edentulous alveolar bone. This is most satisfactorily hidden by an acrylic flange.
- Poor oral hygiene or a high caries rate would make it unwise to expensively restore the abutments and provide a fixed prosthesis which is difficult to clean. A denture could compromise a larger number of teeth, and neither replacement is ideal in this instance. However, a carefully designed partial denture is the better option.

If the patient opted for a removable prosthesis, what designs would you consider?

In this bounded saddle situation a metal-based tooth-supported design is ideal. Both abutment teeth would require a rest seat preparation and one abutment tooth would require a clasp. A palatal connector would be required but need not cover the whole palate, provided sufficient rigidity can be achieved to prevent distortion (which usually occurs out of the mouth). A second clasp on the opposite side would provide sufficient retention.

A mucosa-supported acrylic denture with minimal coverage of the palatal gingival tissues is possible. However this would be difficult to design. There are no other edentulous spaces and an Every-type design would not be possible.

Should the study models be mounted on an articulator to make the bridge?

Properly articulated models mounted with the use of a facebow are essential when a bridge:

- involves many teeth
- changes the anterior guidance
- includes occlusal surfaces involved in guidance
- increases the vertical dimension.

In general an articulator can be helpful when planning and making posterior crowns or bridges on patients who have a class II division 1 incisal relationship and anterior crowns and bridges on patients with a class II division 2 incisal relationship. The choice of articulator will depend on the clinician's preference, but in most cases with straightforward restorations a semiadjustable articulator is satisfactory. For simple crowns and bridges when the guidance is straightforward, such as the present case, either hand-held models or a simple hinge articulator are satisfactory.

What is the ideal design of minimal preparation bridge?

The ideal design of bridge varies with the site of the edentulous space. Various possibilities are shown in Figure 28.2. In the upper anterior region a simple cantilever design lasts longest. In the lower anterior region a fixed–fixed design is usually more dependable because the surface area of enamel on lower incisors is insufficient to support a simple cantilever design. In this situation, a simple cantilever using the molar as a retainer or fixed–fixed or fixed–movable designs are possible.

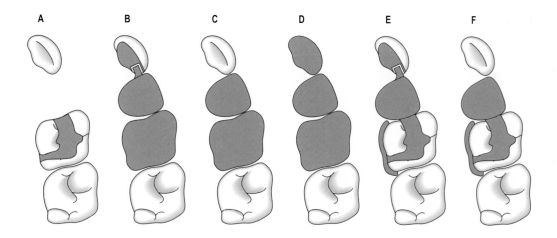

| A | B | C | D | E | F |

Fig. 28.2 Possible bridge designs. The gap can be left and provided overeruption of the opposing teeth does not occur, the existing situation would be stable (A). A possible fixed–movable design (B) would be a minor retainer covering part of the canine and secured to the tooth with an adhesive cement and a conventionally prepared full coverage retainer on the molar. The molar can be conventionally prepared for a full coverage restoration, either for a simple cantilever (C), or in addition the canine can be prepared producing a fixed–fixed design (D). A minimal preparation bridge is also possible. The existing restoration can be partly removed to secure the retainer, and the canine can be either included in a fixed–movable design (E) or avoided to produce a simple cantilever design (F).

In this case a simple cantilever design was selected. The completed bridge is shown in Figures 28.3 and 28.4. To maximize the rigidity of the retainer and increase the surface area of enamel available for bonding, the existing amalgam restoration in the molar was removed and the cavity incorporated into the design. A minimum of 1 mm retainer thickness is required for rigidity, and including the existing cavity into the thickness provides a significant increase in rigidity, reducing flexion and reducing the risk of failure of the bond.

The retainer should cover as much tooth tissue as possible to maximize surface area for bonding. Metal should be wrapped around the abutment tooth as far as possible without encroaching on the contact point. The prepared area should be either within enamel or just into dentine. Modern luting cements bond to dentine and placing part of the preparation in dentine reduces the reliance on the enamel bond. Including the existing cavity also helps, by providing a dentine surface for bonding. The pontic is usually made of porcelain bonded to the metal.

■ *What would you do if the bridge fails through debonding?*

If the bridge decements shortly after placement, it is acceptable to recement the bridge and ensure that there is no occlusal interference. If the problem persists, a conventional bridge would then be indicated, probably using the same abutment teeth for conventional crowns.

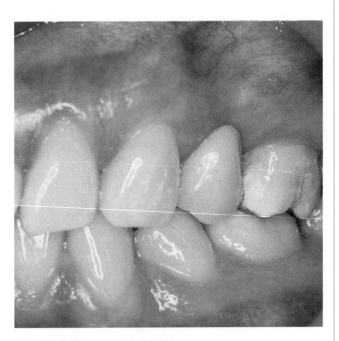

Fig. 28.3 The completed bridge.

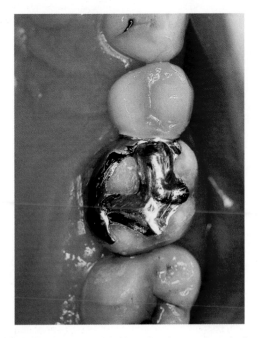

Fig. 28.4 The completed bridge showing retainer design.

CASE 29

Management of anticoagulation

Summary

A 60-year-old man presents to you in your general dental practice requiring a dental extraction. He is taking oral anticoagulants. How will you deal with his extraction?

HISTORY

Complaint

The patient has a broken down upper first molar which is tender on biting. The patient points directly at the tooth and requests extraction.

History of complaint

The tooth has been root-filled and crowned, but is tender to percussion. There have been several episodes of similar pain in the past year. The crown has been lost from the tooth.

Medical history

The patient reports that he had rheumatic fever as a child and as a result of cardiac valve damage he received a prosthetic heart valve 7 years ago. He is taking warfarin (9 mg daily) and co-amilofruse (amiloride/frusemide diuretic combination; 2 tablets daily). The patient carries an anticoagulation card from his local clinic showing that his INR (International Normalized Ratio) prothrombin time is usually between 3.5 and 4.5. It was last checked 10 days ago when it was 3.9.

■ *Would antibiotic cover be required for extraction? If so, what antibiotic would you give?*

Yes, a prosthetic heart valve is a high risk factor for the development of infective endocarditis. The recommended antibiotic cover in this situation is 3 g of amoxycillin taken orally 1 hour prior to the extraction. This assumes the patient is not allergic to penicillin and has not had more than one other dose of penicillin in the past month.

■ *How does warfarin work and how is anticoagulation monitored?*

Warfarin is a vitamin K antagonist. It prevents the liver from utilizing vitamin K to make clotting factors II, VII, IX and X. The patient is usually under the care of an anticoagulation clinic,

although some patients are monitored by their GP. Blood tests are performed regularly and the results and drug doses are recorded in a yellow book that the patient should always carry.

■ *What is the INR test, what is its normal therapeutic range and how should the result be interpreted?*

The International Normalized Ratio is a standardized prothrombin time test. The result is the ratio of the patient's prothrombin time to that of a standardized control and measures the effectiveness of the extrinsic and common pathways of blood coagulation, i.e. those most affected by warfarin. The therapeutic range for patients who have had deep vein thrombosis or pulmonary embolism is 2.5–3.5. For patients with a prosthetic heart valve it is 3.5–4.5, at the top of the therapeutic range.

In theory the INR is a standardized test using an internationally accepted standard. Unfortunately, in practice accurate standardization of the INR is often not possible, and small changes in the decimal places of the result cannot be relied upon to reflect small changes in anticoagulation. The test should be regarded as an estimate of anticoagulation rather than an accurate measure.

EXAMINATION

Extraoral examination

No lymphadenopathy is present and the extraoral examination reveals no abnormalities. However, a large bruise is apparent on the patient's right forearm, consistent with the degree of anticoagulation.

Intraoral examination

The patient has a number of teeth with large restorations and several crowned teeth. His periodontal condition and oral hygiene are relatively good with only small amounts of detectable interdental plaque.

The upper first molar tooth is broken down. Root-filling material can be seen in the open pulp chamber and much of the root surface is carious. The tooth is tender to percussion. The second premolar is not tender to percussion but produces a dull percussive note. No sinus is present. Periodontal probing cannot be carried out without antibiotic cover, but the periodontal condition seems reasonable and there seems to be no significant bone loss.

There is caries around the distal margin of a crown on the first premolar.

INVESTIGATIONS

■ *What investigations are required and why?*

The premolars and molars should be checked for vitality. The first premolar is vital but both second premolar and first molar do not respond to testing with an electric pulp tester.

A radiograph is required in order to decide whether the molar is restorable, that is, to gauge the extent of caries and determine the success of the root filling. If extraction turns out to be required, a radiograph will be necessary to assess the difficulty of the extraction. This is particularly important in a patient who may suffer prolonged bleeding. A periapical view is the ideal view.

■ *The periapical view is shown in Figure 29.1. What does it show?*

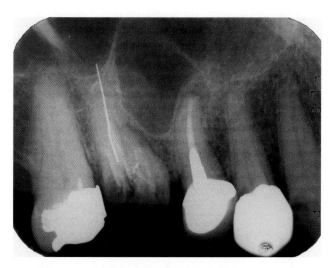

Fig. 29.1 Periapical radiograph of the upper first molar.

The first permanent molar is extensively carious. A root filling is present but only one gutta percha or silver point is visible, in the palatal canal. It extends beyond the apex by approximately 2 mm. The buccal roots are not clearly visible but appear to contain no root filling. The overextended root filling lies close to the antrum and the antrum extends down between the roots of the first molar and second premolar. There is no apical radiolucency. The second premolar is also root-filled. The root filling appears to stop just short of the anatomical apex at an appropriate point but a small apical radiolucency is present, surrounded by the lamina dura of the tooth socket. The caries below the crown on the first premolar is visible and the second molar contains a large pinned amalgam.

DIAGNOSIS

■ *What is your diagnosis? Explain your diagnosis.*

The patient's pain is caused by periapical periodontitis of the first permanent molar.

The patient points clearly to this tooth as the cause of his pain. This and the tenderness on percussion indicate inflammation of the periodontal ligament and the overfilled root canal provides a likely cause. No radiolucency is shown on the radiograph. However, none is required for diagnosis in the presence of typical signs and symptoms. There may be either only a small apical lesion or one on the apices of the buccal roots or in the trifurcation, both of which are superimposed on the film.

The second premolar has an unsuccessful root filling and granuloma or a small radicular cyst at the apex. However, it is not tender to percussion and is not felt as the cause by the patient. The first premolar is vital and the caries would

produce pain of pulpitis type without tenderness on biting or percussion.

TREATMENT

■ *What treatment would you recommend?*

The primary consideration should be that the patient is at risk of infective endocarditis and potential sources of infection should be eradicated. The first molar cannot be restored without another root filling and extensive preparation. The patient prefers extraction and this is the appropriate course of action. The first premolar is more problematic. It is apparently symptom-free and the apical granuloma has probably been present for some time. This lesion is a further potential source of infection and it must be eliminated, either by extraction or another root filling. The success of the new root filling must be monitored to ensure that it is successful, and if not either apicectomy or extraction will need to be considered. Elements of this treatment would require antibiotic cover and/or adjustment of anticoagulation, and so these items must be incorporated into a complete treatment plan which takes the rest of the dentition into account.

■ *Is the extraction of the first molar likely to be straightforward?*

No. The tooth is broken down and root-filled and there is little or no bone loss from periodontitis. It will be difficult to grasp with forceps and may be brittle. The roots extend close to the antrum and there is a risk of creating a surgical oroantral fistula.

A simple forceps extraction might turn out to be possible, but extraction may well require a mucoperiosteal flap and bone removal. A simple forceps extraction would be preferable in an anticoagulated patient because bleeding is more easily controlled when it is limited to a socket and surrounding gingiva. A surgical extraction would be less traumatic overall and separating the roots and elevating them singly would reduce the chances of creating an oroantral fistula.

■ *Would you expect this patient to suffer prolonged bleeding after a dental extraction?*

Yes, definitely, and, if untreated, such bleeding could require hospital admission. Untreated prolonged haemorrhage could be fatal. The patient will require adjustment in his warfarin dose in order to reduce the INR.

■ *To what level must the INR be reduced for the performance of minor oral surgery?*

The INR must be reduced for procedures where prolonged bleeding may be of concern, such as intramuscular injections, minor surgery and dental extraction (see Table 29.1.)

For more major surgery the patient would need to be switched from warfarin to heparin. Heparin has a half life of a few hours and its effects are more readily reversed in an emergency.

Table 29.1 Acceptable INRs for various procedures

Procedure	Acceptable INR
Infiltration anaesthesia	<4.5
ID block	<2.5
Simple extraction / uncomplicated surgical extraction	<2.5
Soft tissue surgery	<2.5

■ *How recently should the last INR test have been done?*

A result from the previous day reflects the bleeding tendency, provided the anticoagulation is stable. However, if the INR result on the patient's anticoagulation record card fluctuates without change in dose, only a test performed on the day of treatment should be accepted. If there has been no recent test, one should be requested, or alternatively the appointment may be postponed until the next test result is available.

■ *How would you go about reducing the warfarin dosage?*

If the ratio is too high the patient's warfarin dose will require alteration. *Consultation with the medical practitioner responsible for anticoagulation (usually a haematologist) is mandatory.* After consultation, the patient would normally take a lower dose of warfarin (but not stop it), and an INR test can be performed on the day of the procedure to confirm that the INR is acceptable.

Warfarin doses must be taken at the same time each day, and this is usually in the evening. Warfarin should be restarted in the evening of the day of the procedure.

In this case the warfarin dose was reduced and the INR fell to 2.4. The tooth was extracted and the socket sutured under antibiotic cover.

■ *What additional precautions might you take to ensure haemostasis and reduce the chances of postoperative bleeding?*

In general, warfarin is associated with oozing of blood from soft tissues rather than bleeding from bone. Bleeding is most readily reduced by placing a single interrupted or mattress suture across the mouth of the socket to exert gentle pressure on the gingiva. In the event of bleeding from bone, Whitehead's varnish or a Surgicel pack may be placed but this is rarely necessary.

If there is severe periodontitis then treating this first, even if only around a few teeth, much reduces postoperative bleeding.

Following extraction you place a single suture and achieve haemostasis after a slightly prolonged period.

■ *The patient returns 3 hours later indicating that bleeding has continued throughout most of this period. Why has bleeding restarted?*

Bleeding in the immediate postoperative period is stopped by platelet plugs forming in the vessels. This mechanism is unaffected by warfarin which inhibits only coagulation. After the initial haemostasis, coagulation fails to consolidate the platelet plugs. When the vasoconstrictor in the local anaesthetic wears off, there is a period of hyperaemia as a result of inflammation and bleeding starts again.

■ *How would you manage this postextraction bleeding?*

Initially, check that the socket is only oozing as rapid bleeding would necessitate immediate measures. Then take a history and assess the degree of blood loss which, to the patient (and sometimes the dentist), always seems worse than it actually is. Examine the patient using a good light and suction to remove the poorly formed blood clots and identify the bleeding area. Apply pressure by getting the patient to bite upon a gauze swab shaped to press *only* onto the socket.

After 10 minutes continuous pressure, remove the swab and review the bleeding. If only the soft tissue is bleeding, pressure may be all that is required and the patient can be instructed to repeat the procedure if required. However, if there is still bleeding and the socket has been sutured, as in this case, bleeding may be arising from the bone. Open the socket and pack it with Surgicel or Whitehead's varnish which is almost always effective. Resuture the socket. Bone wax should only be used if this fails because bone wax delays healing in the longer term. Then replace sutures over the pack to provide pressure to the gingival margins and to keep the pack firmly in the socket.

Reassure the patient, who is often very worried and well aware of the problems of their anticoagulation treatment. Observe for 15–30 minutes and reinforce normal postoperative instructions. It is emphasized that the patient must not rinse until the next day. It is unlikely that these measures will fail.

■ *What would you do if these steps did fail?*

In a practice setting the patient should be transferred to a hospital casualty or specialist unit, or their anticoagulation clinic. This should be arranged speedily and the patient will require an escort. There the INR and platelet count would be checked. Antifibrinolytics, such as aprotinin and tranexamic acid can be used in conjunction with packing and suturing. If the bleeding persists the patient will need to be admitted for reversal of the anticoagulation by infusion of fresh frozen plasma. Vitamin K injections will not reverse the action of the warfarin for 12 hours and are not effective in such emergency situations.

■ *What would you do if there were tachycardia and lowered blood pressure?*

This would indicate significant blood loss and, as above, the patient should be speedily admitted to hospital for intravenous fluids to prevent circulatory collapse.

■ *Does treatment to stop bleeding require administration of a further dose of antibiotic cover?*

This is a grey area for which there are no clear recommendations. The single dose which has been given will provide cover for 3 hours of routine dental treatment. If bleeding can be stopped with pressure or a suture alone, no additional cover is warranted. However, if a longer time had elapsed and the socket is to be opened, a second dose is, in theory, necessary. A half dose might provide sufficient additional antibiotic to maintain an adequate blood level for a further hour but this course of action would have to be agreed by the patient's cardiologist. If more than 4 hours had elapsed, a further 3 g of amoxycillin would be required under the current recommendations. This assumes the patient had not had another course or dose of any penicillin drug in the past month. If they had, a change of drug to clindamycin would be required.

In terms of risk assessment, the value of any second dose is extremely small; the extraction would have caused a much greater bacteraemia than suturing the socket. It is accepted that there is little proven benefit from antibiotic prophylaxis and the risk of a coagulation complication from reducing the warfarin dose is probably greater than the risk of endocarditis, even in a patient with a prosthetic heart valve.

■ *Warfarin interacts with a variety of other drugs. Which drugs that might be prescribed in dental practice can affect warfarin anticoagulation?*

Drugs inducing liver enzymes
Nonsteroidal anti-inflammatory drugs
Antibiotics, including erythromycin, metronidazole, tetracyclines and penicillins
Fluconazole, ketoconazole and miconazole (including topical preparations)

In all cases there is increased anticoagulation and a risk of bleeding. Aspirin and related drugs also increase the risk of bleeding, not by interaction but through their separate antiplatelet activity. Discussion with the patient's anticoagulation clinic would be prudent if any of these drugs are required.

A white patch on the tongue

Summary
A 52-year-old woman has a white patch on her tongue. Make a diagnosis and decide on appropriate treatment.

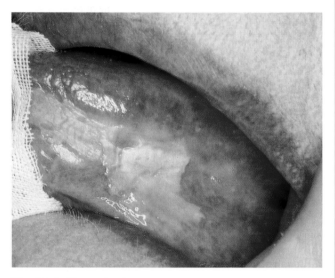

Fig. 30.1 The patient's tongue.

HISTORY

Complaint
The patient has no complaint.

History of complaint
You have just noticed the lesion in a patient attending for the first time for several years. There is no written record of the white patch in her notes. The patient had noticed the lesion but has ignored it. She thinks it has probably been there for several years.

Medical history
The patient is otherwise fit and well. She smokes 4 cigarettes a day and drinks 4–8 units of alcohol each week.

EXAMINATION

Extraoral examination
No lymph nodes are palpable in the neck and there are no abnormal findings on extraoral examination.

Intraoral examination
Apart from this lesion, the remainder of the oral mucosa is normal.

■ *The appearance of the lesion is shown in Figure 30.1. What do you see?*

There is a flat and homogeneous white patch on the left lateral border and ventral tongue mucosa. It is well defined and varies slightly in whiteness.

If you were able to feel the lesion you would find that it is soft and feels no different from the surrounding mucosa.

DIFFERENTIAL DIAGNOSIS

■ *What are the common or important white patches in the mouth? How are they caused?*

Almost all oral white patches are caused by increased keratinization of the epithelium. Keratin absorbs water and appears white, brighter white where it is thicker. The exception is a chemical burn where the white surface layer is caused by necrosis or ulceration.

Type of lesion	White lesion(s)
Normal mucosal variants	Leukoedema Fordyce spots/granules
Inherited epithelial disorders	White sponge naevus Pachyonychia congenita
Traumatic lesions	Frictional keratosis Chemical burn Cheek and tongue biting
Infections	Thrush (acute hyperplastic candidiasis) Chronic hyperplastic candidiasis (candidal *leukoplakia*) Chronic mucocutaneous candidiasis Hairy leukoplakia Syphilitic leukoplakia
Lichen planus and similar conditions	Lichen planus Lichenoid reaction (topical and systemic) Lupus erythematosus
Unknown or smoking-related	Idiopathic keratosis (*leukoplakia*), *including:* Homogeneous leukoplakia Verrucous/nodular leukoplakia Sublingual keratosis Smoker's keratosis Speckled leukoplakia Stomatitis nicotina (smoker's palate)
Neoplastic	Squamous cell carcinoma

■ *Which lesions would you include in the differential diagnosis for the current lesion?*

Likely diagnoses:
— Idiopathic white patch (*leukoplakia*)

Sublingual keratosis
Smoker's keratosis
— Frictional keratosis.

Less likely diagnoses:
— Chronic hyperplastic candidiasis
— Lichen planus or lichenoid reaction
— Tongue biting
— Squamous cell carcinoma.

■ *What is a leukoplakia?*

The literal meaning of leukoplakia is white patch. The term is correctly defined as a white patch which cannot be characterized as any other lesion. It can only be used correctly after all possible known causes have been eliminated, using whatever investigations are required. Unfortunately the term leukoplakia is often used very loosely in a clinical context, either for a white patch of any cause or for the small minority of white patches which have a risk of malignant transformation. This has led to great confusion. Now that the term has also been incorporated into the names of several lesions for which the cause is known (such as candidal leukoplakia, hairy leukoplakia and syphilitic leukoplakia) the term has become so inconsistently used as to be unhelpful.

■ *Justify your differential diagnosis.*

Idiopathic white patch. Although many causes of well defined white patches are known, the largest single group is that for which no cause can be identified. This is therefore a likely diagnosis and there are no clinical features which suggest a specific cause for the present lesion. The group of idiopathic white patches includes some more specific terms which might be applied to this lesion.
• **Sublingual keratosis** is a white patch affecting the floor of the mouth or ventral tongue and lesions here are considered to have a high risk of malignant transformation. The typical lesion is bilateral and may be extensive in the floor of the mouth, often with a wrinkled surface of 'ebbing tide' parallel corrugations. However, sublingual keratosis is defined only by its site and any white patch affecting the ventral tongue or floor of mouth could be termed a sublingual keratosis. The present lesion does include ventral tongue mucosa.
• **Smoker's keratosis** is a white patch in the mouth of a smoker for which no other cause can be found. The type of lesion usually called smoker's keratosis is a flat homogeneous white patch, sometimes with a finely wrinkled surface, on nonkeratinized mucosa. The smoking is assumed to be the cause, though there is rarely any evidence to support this unless the lesion arises where a pipe or cigarette is habitually held. This patient's lesion could be called a smoker's keratosis but this is not a particularly useful label and does not imply that it should be treated any differently from an idiopathic white patch. Smoker's palate (stomatitis nicotina) is a separate condition and is discussed below.

Frictional keratosis is common along the occlusal line, on edentulous alveolar ridges and the lateral tongue. It may be associated with sharp teeth or restoration(s) and be unilateral or bilateral. Frictional keratosis usually merges gradually with the surrounding normal mucosa and is not as sharply defined as the present lesion. Tongue biting also causes keratosis but the surface is often shredded and there may be similar lesions on the buccal mucosa, usually just behind the commissure. Unless lesions are associated with clear evidence of habitual biting, sharp teeth, or resolve on removing a cause, it can be very difficult to identify them from their clinical appearance. Frictional keratosis should be included in the differential diagnosis.

Chronic hyperplastic candidiasis causes white plaques, sometimes called candidal leukoplakia. These arise most commonly on the postcommissural buccal mucosa and dorsal tongue and may be associated with red areas. This lesion is more common in smokers. Unless the site is typical it is almost impossible to make the diagnosis clinically. Biopsy or resolution on antifungal treatment are the most useful investigations. The present lesion is not typical, but this cause cannot be confidently excluded on clinical grounds.

Lichen planus and lichenoid reactions may cause homogeneous white patches. This more unusual presentation seems to be more common in smokers and it is not at all clear whether these so-called *plaque-type lichen planus* lesions are a genuine presentation of lichen planus or are smoking-induced. To be sure of the diagnosis it is desirable to find evidence of more typical lichen planus elsewhere, either on the skin, the buccal mucosa or in the form of desquamative gingivitis. There is no evidence to suggest that the current lesion is caused by lichen planus but the plaque type cannot be completely excluded on clinical grounds alone.

Squamous cell carcinoma. This diagnosis must be included for any white patch in the mouth without an identified cause. The chances of this particular lesion being malignant appear low. Although it is in a high risk site, it is a flat homogeneous lesion without ulceration, red areas, speckling or induration. The patient is a light smoker and is in the risk age group for squamous carcinoma. Though very unlikely, *this just might be a carcinoma.*

■ *Which white lesions have you excluded? Explain why.*

• *Leukoedema* and patches of *Fordyce spots* (sebaceous glands) are normal mucosal variants which affect primarily the buccal mucosa. Leukoedema causes a milky white appearance and is usually seen in those of negroid racial stock. Fordyce spots are sebaceous glands. They occasionally form clusters which resemble plaques but have a slightly yellow appearance and individual glands are usually visible within the lesion. Both are present from childhood and neither affect the lateral tongue.
• *White sponge naevus* and *pachyonychia congenita* are examples of rare inherited conditions which cause diffuse keratosis or multiple discrete white patches on the mucosa. These possibilities are excluded by the localized extent of the lesion, age of onset and the absence of other skin or nail abnormalities and family history.

- *An aspirin burn* or other form of chemical trauma is unlikely. This results from application of aspirin directly to the mucosa, usually in response to toothache. Lesions are mostly in the buccal sulcus and affect mucosa on both sides of the site where the tablet was placed. This is an unlikely possibility and may be readily excluded by direct questioning.
- *Thrush* affects larger areas of the mucosa, at least parts of the lesion may be wiped off and the underlying mucosa is inflamed. Chronic candidiasis could cause the present lesion and is discussed above.
- *Hairy leukoplakia* usually forms bilateral white lesions along the lateral border of the tongue in immunosuppressed patients. While the possibility of an undiagnosed immunosuppression, particularly from HIV infection, cannot be excluded, the appearances are not typical of hairy leukoplakia. Lesions remain limited to the lateral tongue in almost all cases.
- *Syphilitic leukoplakia* may also be readily excluded, being now of only historical interest. The patient must have tertiary syphilis and the site of the white patches is the dorsum of the tongue.
- *Smoker's palate* or *stomatitis nicotina* may be excluded because it affects only the hard palate of pipe, cigar and heavy cigarette smokers.

INVESTIGATIONS

■ *Should a biopsy be performed? Explain why.*

Yes. As a general rule, all white lesions in the mouth merit biopsy. Completely typical keratotic lichen planus and typical frictional keratoses are considered exceptions to this rule by some authorities, but this would only be acceptable if the clinician were very experienced in the diagnosis of oral white lesions. Even those with extensive experience can be deceived occasionally by a carcinoma which appears to be an innocuous white lesion.

The reasons for performing biopsy are:
- To exclude/confirm squamous cell carcinoma.
- If not malignant, to determine whether dysplasia is present.
- To identify chronic candidal infection if present.
- To help identify specific conditions and cause(s) for the lesion.

■ *Is this lesion suitable for biopsy in general dental practice? Explain why.*

Yes. The final decision will depend on your experience and confidence, but there is no reason why this biopsy should not be performed in general dental practice.

■ *What lesions should emphatically not be subjected to biopsy in general dental practice?*

Biopsy of the following mucosal lesions would not be appropriate in general dental practice, though they might be performed by those with more specialized experience.

Lesion	Reason
Any lesion which shows clinical features suggesting malignancy	These should be sampled by the person or team who will manage the patient's care. If you perform a biopsy you are taking upon yourself the responsibility of telling the patient the diagnosis. Refer the patient to a hospital for urgent opinion and biopsy. See also case 31.
Lesions which will require hospital care or treatment once the diagnosis is made	Comprehensive care for the patient is improved when investigation, diagnosis and treatment are carried out in an integrated fashion.
Haemangiomas and other vascular lesions	These may bleed excessively.
Lesions on the posterior soft palate or fauces	Tearing of the thin mucosa and retching make wound closure difficult.
Inaccessible lesions	If you cannot guarantee to remove an ideal specimen refer the patient. Inadequate specimens provide no benefit for the patient.
Swellings of possible minor salivary gland origin other than mucocoeles	There is a significant risk that these lesions may be neoplasms and about half will be malignant.

Only the first two reasons might apply to this lesion and, as noted above, the lesion has no features to suggest malignancy, is readily accessible and easily anaesthetized. It is representative of the large majority of white patches found in the population which have a very low risk of malignant change and are ideal for biopsy in general practice.

■ *What features of a white patch might indicate malignancy and contraindicate biopsy in practice?*

- Associated red areas
- Speckled areas
- Ulceration, especially if chronic
- Induration
- Enlarged lymph nodes draining the site
- Lesion in a high risk site.

■ *How much would you remove and from where?*

The ideal biopsy sample of mucosa to assess a white patch or mucosal condition is approximately 10 mm long and 4–5 mm wide. The sample should extend to muscle and provide sufficient deep tissue to support the epithelial sample and for the pathologist to inspect microscopically. In the lateral tongue this is only 2–3 mm depth because the muscle lies near the surface. In buccal mucosa the ideal depth is slightly more, up to 5 mm. If a lesion is suspected to extend deeply then a thicker sample will be required. This size of sample is readily removed, the wound easily closed, and healing is quick and without significant symptoms.

The site sampled should comprise mostly the lesion but with a part of the margin and some adjacent normal mucosa. In a higher risk lesion any suspicious areas (see list above) would be included. If several such areas were present, multiple samples might be required.

■ *The biopsy specimen is required to assess dysplasia. What is meant by dysplasia?*

Dysplasia means abnormal growth and can be used in different senses. Conditions termed dysplastic include developmental disturbances (such as ectodermal dysplasia), benign self-limiting overgrowths (such as fibrous dysplasia) and potentially malignant epithelial lesions. When applied to oral white or red patches, dysplasia means the microscopic changes which indicate a risk of malignant transformation.

■ *What are the features of epithelial dysplasia?*

Dysplasia is recognized by combinations of the following histological features:

Growth abnormality	Detected by presence of
Failure to form an organized epithelial layer	No well defined basal cell, prickle and squamous cell layers (and keratin layer if present) Increased number of layers of basal cells Drop-shaped rete processes Loss of polarity of the cells: vertically orientated rather than flattening towards the surface Loss of cohesion between cells
Disordered maturation and differentiation of single cells	Change in keratin pattern Keratinization of single cells or clusters of cells deep in the epithelium rather than at the surface Cells of bizarre shape (cytoplasmic pleomorphism)
Abnormalities of cell nuclei	Darkly staining nuclei (hyperchromatism) Nuclei of varying sizes (anisonucleosis) Cells with bizarre nuclei (nuclear pleomorphism)
Abnormal growth regulation	Increased numbers of mitoses Mitoses in suprabasal cells Abnormal mitoses

■ *How do these changes differ from the histological changes seen in squamous carcinoma?*

Many, if not all, of these features are usually seen in squamous carcinomas. Carcinoma differs from dysplasia because it invades the underlying tissues, usually as separate islands and strands of epithelium, and may metastasize to distant sites.

■ *How is dysplasia assessed?*

The scoring of dysplasia is extremely difficult, not very reproducible and requires experience. Most pathologists divide dysplastic lesions into categories of mild, moderate and severe. Severe dysplasia is sometimes called *carcinoma in situ.*

With increasing severity of dysplasia there is increasing risk of malignant transformation. Although dysplasia is the best indicator of the risk of development of malignancy, the relationship between the two is complex. Severe dysplasia nearly always indicates a relatively high risk, but carcinoma will occasionally develop in a white lesion which shows minimal dysplasia.

■ *Does dysplasia always progress?*

No. Dysplasia does not always progress and in some cases it may regress. Dysplasia indicates increased potential to become malignant but does not necessarily mean that any lesion will eventually do so.

■ *The histological features of the lesion are shown in Figure 30.2. What do you see and how do you interpret the changes?*

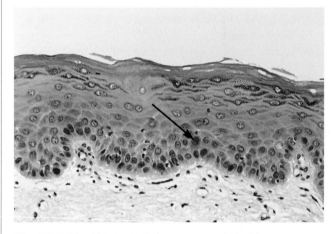

Fig. 30.2 The histological appearances of the biopsy sample.

The surface is covered by a regular orthokeratinized stratified squamous epithelium. The basement membrane is almost flat with a few short dermal papillae extending up into the epithelium. The epithelium is abnormal for either lateral border or ventral tongue, neither of which show even orthokeratosis.

There are minimal signs of dysplasia. The epithelium shows good stratification with well organized basal, prickle cell, granular cell and keratin layers, each composed of cells at the same stage of maturation. The basal cell layer is slightly disorganized. Instead of a well defined single layer of small dark cells there is a slightly irregular layer of cells whose nuclei vary a little in size and staining intensity. Near the centre there is one darkly staining cell in a suprabasal position (arrowed). No candida was found in a section stained with PAS stain.

The changes of abnormal keratinization and slight basal cell irregularity are not very marked. The epithelial cells form a well organized epithelium; there are only occasional abnormal single cells, minimal nuclear abnormalities and no evidence of increased growth. These signs might be graded as either nondysplastic or mildly dysplastic depending on the pathologist. The final diagnosis given in this case was keratosis with mild dysplasia.

Feature	Risk of malignant transformation
Dysplasia	The degree of dysplasia is the best predictor and it may change, either progressing or regressing, with time.
Site	White lesions in the floor of mouth, posterior and lateral tongue and retromolar area carry the highest risk. Those on the hard palate and dorsum of tongue carry no significant risk. This distribution matches the distribution of oral squamous cell carcinoma.
Colour	Development of red areas carries a high risk and is usually associated with severe dysplasia histologically.
Surface	Development of verrucous or nodular areas.
Tobacco use	Smoking indicates increased risk. However, smoking also causes many white patches with no dysplasia and so, statistically, patches in nonsmokers carry an even higher risk.
Age	The risk of malignant transformation rises with age.
Sex	Female patients are at higher risk (despite the fact that oral carcinoma is commoner in men).
Size	Larger lesions have a higher risk of malignant transformation.
Duration	Patches present for a longer time have a higher risk of malignant transformation.
Family history of carcinoma in upper aerodigestive tract	Indicates increased risk.
Candidal infection in presence of dysplasia	Indicates a small increase in risk.
Change in clinical appearance	Changes apart from colour, such as size, nodularity or development of a verrucous surface indicate a higher risk.
Underlying conditions	Conditions which predispose to oral carcinoma, such as submucous fibrosis, raise the relative risk of malignant transformation.

DIAGNOSIS

■ *What is the final diagnosis? Is this a risk lesion for malignant transformation?*

The diagnosis is idiopathic white patch (or keratosis) with mild dysplasia. This is a risk lesion for malignant transformation.

TREATMENT

■ *What treatment is indicated?*

The following principles of treatment apply to all idiopathic keratoses. The patient should stop smoking and moderate their alcohol intake. If candidal infection had been detected it should be treated and checked for recurrence periodically. In this case, and others in which dysplasia is mild or absent, it is appropriate to monitor the lesion closely for changes in appearance, initially at 3-monthly intervals and extending to annual review provided the lesion does not change significantly. The aim is to detect any change in the severity of dysplasia or malignant transformation and this may require biopsy from time to time, depending on the changes noted. Photographic or digital images aid recognition of changes and are a valuable adjunct to the long-term review of white lesions.

Lesions with moderate or severe dysplasia may be excised, ablated by laser or treated with topical chemotherapeutic agents such as bleomycin. Occasionally patches are too large to treat in these ways and the only option is to monitor to detect malignant transformation as early as possible.

In addition it is important to remember that dysplasia probably affects all mucosa exposed to tobacco smoke and alcohol. There is a risk of carcinoma arising in the pharynx and respiratory tract and symptoms from these areas indicate a need for endoscopy.

PROGNOSIS

■ *What features would indicate that a white patch might become malignant over the coming years?*

See Table above.

In this case the lesion remained unchanged and the patient was reviewed at 3-monthly intervals for 1 year, 6-monthly intervals for 2 years and she continues under annual review. Four years after presentation a second biopsy was performed and the degree of dysplasia was still mild. Excision has been considered because the lesion is relatively accessible and in a high risk site for carcinoma, but has not been carried out because the dysplasia remains mild and the patient prefers not to have surgery. She keeps her patch under close observation, returning for appointments if she feels it has changed.

CASE 31

Another white patch on the tongue

Summary
A 39-year-old woman has a white patch on the lateral margin of her tongue. What is the cause and what are the treatment options?

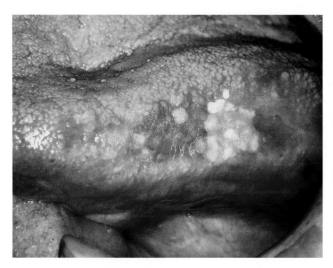

Fig. 31.1 The patient's tongue.

HISTORY

Complaint
The patient has no symptoms.

History of complaint
The patient is an infrequent dental attender and has not been to the dentist for at least 5 years. Following an oral cancer awareness week she inspected her mouth and became nervous about her tongue. She would like it checked.

Medical history
She has had cervical dysplasia treated in the previous year by cone biopsy and this has left her very worried about cancer. She is otherwise fit and well.

She has smoked 40 cigarettes daily since the age of 18 years and drinks 14 units of alcohol per week as spirits.

EXAMINATION

Extraoral examination
She seems a healthy woman with no obvious skin, nail or eye lesions present on visible skin. No lymph nodes are palpable in the neck.

Intraoral examination
The oral mucosa appears normal, except for the tongue which is shown in Figure 31.1.

■ *Describe the appearance of the tongue lesion.*

Site	Right lateral border of tongue
Size	1 × 3 cm approximately
Shape	Ill defined ellipse
Colour	Mixture of white and red components
Surface	Appears nodular or irregular

Palpation reveals the lesion to be firmer than the adjacent mucosa. The white component of the area cannot be rubbed away. The tongue is freely mobile.

DIFFERENTIAL DIAGNOSIS

■ *What are the causes of mixed red and white patches in the mouth?*

The causes of white patches are discussed more fully in case 30. Several causes may also be associated with red areas.

Cause	Red and white lesion(s)
Trauma	Chemical burn Cheek biting
Infection	Thrush (acute hyperplastic candidiasis) Chronic hyperplastic candidiasis (candidal *leukoplakia*)
Lichen planus and similar conditions	Lichen planus Lichenoid reaction (topical and systemic) Lupus erythematosus
Idiopathic or smoking	Idiopathic keratosis (*leukoplakia*) *including*: Sublingual keratosis Smoker's keratosis Speckled leukoplakia Stomatitis nicotina (smoker's palate)
Neoplasia	Squamous cell carcinoma

■ *Which of the above lesions would you include in the differential diagnosis for this particular lesion?*

1. Squamous cell carcinoma
2. Idiopathic white patch with or without dysplasia including speckled leukoplakia
3. Chronic hyperplastic candidiasis
4. Lichenoid reaction.

■ *Justify this differential diagnosis.*

The most important consideration in differential diagnosis for all oral white patches is that squamous carcinoma or a premalignant lesion may be the cause. This is especially so when lesions are red and white or speckled.

Squamous carcinoma is a likely diagnosis and the most significant diagnosis. Although this patient is young for a squamous carcinoma, cases are seen in the fourth decade of life and the incidence in younger patients appears to be increasing both in the UK and elsewhere. The patient drinks and smokes heavily and these are the main risk factors for oral squamous cell carcinoma. She drinks 14 units of alcohol per week (maximum recommended intake 14 units female, 21 units male). These maximum intakes are considered 'safe' in terms of cardiovascular disease risk and no safe limit is recognized for the oral mucosa. There is no safe intake for tobacco and the combined relative risk for this patient to develop carcinoma is at least 5–10 times higher than for a non-smoker or occasional drinker. The presence of the lesion in a high-risk site, its speckled appearance and association with smoking are very worrying regardless of the patient's age. This lesion should be considered a carcinoma until proved otherwise.

A premalignant lesion would be the next most likely diagnosis. Option 2 in the differential diagnosis covers all white patches of unknown aetiology, some of which carry a risk of malignant transformation and show dysplasia on microscopic examination. The risk of malignant transformation is higher in those with a red component which may be either a speckled area or in a separate, usually adjacent, site. The risk factors are the same as those for carcinoma, and if this lesion is not a carcinoma it is almost certainly premalignant.

■ *Which lesions are less likely possibilities? Explain why.*

Candidal infection should always be considered as a cause of white patches, particularly when red areas are associated. It is very common. The combination of red and white is most likely to signify thrush (acute hyperplastic candidiasis). However, lesions of thrush are usually more widespread than in the present case and at least some of the white plaques may be removed by rubbing. Chronic hyperplastic candidiasis (candidal *leukoplakia*) forms a discrete white plaque which is sometimes associated with red areas. Although it is normally found on the buccal mucosa and dorsal surface of the tongue, it is a possible diagnosis for the current lesion. It should also be remembered that almost any white patch in the mouth may be susceptible to superinfection by candida simply because of the increased thickness of keratin on the surface of the epithelium. Thus the presence of candidal infection does not preclude an underlying carcinoma, dysplasia or a lichen planus-like condition.

Lichen planus and similar conditions are relatively common causes of intraoral white lesions. Lichen planus, lichenoid reactions and lupus erythematosus are usually readily identifiable by virtue of a presence of lacy white striae,

association with atrophic areas and/or desquamative gingivitis and their symmetrical bilateral distribution. In smokers, both lichen planus and lichenoid reactions may present as discrete white plaques but these *plaque-type* lesions are not usually associated with red areas. Localized single white lesions may also result from topically induced lichenoid reactions such as those to dental restorative materials. However, these are all most unlikely to be responsible for the current lesion because their clinical appearance and distribution are distinct.

■ *What features might indicate that this lesion is already malignant? Which are early and which are late signs?*

Feature	Early	Late
Red or speckled areas	*	*
Nonhealing ulceration	*	*
Rolled everted ulcer margin		*
Induration of surrounding tissues		*
Bleeding from the surface		*
Fixation of the tissues		*
Destruction of adjacent bone		*
Enlarged hard lymph nodes		*
Size	Small carcinomas are probably those which have been diagnosed early but there is great variation in rate of growth and this is only an assumption	
Pain	Unpredictable, often absent, sometimes the presenting complaint	

INVESTIGATIONS

■ *What special investigations are indicated?*

A biopsy is generally considered mandatory for any oral white lesion. This is especially important if no cause is apparent. When malignancy or significant dysplasia is suspected, as in the present case, the biopsy should be performed as soon as possible because early diagnosis is a major factor for successful treatment of oral squamous carcinoma.

■ *Would you perform this biopsy in general practice?*

No, definitely not. Although removing a sample of the tissue is well within the capability of the general practitioner, it would be unwise to do so. The patient will return for the result and practitioners are not usually the appropriate person to break the news of malignant disease. There is also a theoretical risk that biopsy of the wrong site or removal of the whole of a small lesion might compromise subsequent treatment but this is a largely theoretical problem. In a practice environment the patient should be referred urgently, or preferably the same day, to the centre where definitive treatment is likely to be provided. This will allow the most appropriate biopsy to be performed. No other special investigations are indicated at this stage.

■ *Which part of the lesion should be removed for biopsy?*

The specimen should include those areas most likely to be malignant, the red and speckled parts. Some normal tissue should also be included and the sample should be about 1 cm long, 4–5 mm wide, and an even depth including underlying muscle. Larger malignancies are often friable and if the specimen is too small it may disintegrate on removal. No attempt should be made to excise the whole lesion until a diagnosis is obtained.

■ *The biopsy specimen is shown in Figure 31.2. What are the microscopic features and how do you interpret them?*

The lower power view (Fig. 31.2a) shows tongue mucosa with underlying muscle. The overlying epithelium is very irregular and instead of being an even and well organized layer it forms an irregular series of rete processes which penetrate deeply into the underlying tissue. The deepest epithelium is breaking off into apparently separate islands and strands and these extend deeply between muscle bundles. The higher power (Fig. 31.2b) view is taken from the deep surface and shows the deepest epithelium invading muscle. The epithelium is disorganized, with keratin forming in the centre of islands and an irregular darkly stained basal cell layer around the edge. This epithelium has lost its ordered maturation and stratification and is invading the underlying muscle. These features indicate malignancy and the malignant epithelium shows squamous differentiation.

DIAGNOSIS

■ *What is the diagnosis?*

The patient has a squamous cell carcinoma. It is only superficially invasive and probably an early lesion.

TREATMENT

■ *What types of treatment are possible and what is the prognosis?*

The lesion appears to have been diagnosed at a much earlier stage than most oral carcinomas. Treatment may be by radiotherapy (implant or external beam), by surgery or both in combination. The final decision will depend on the results of investigations to stage the carcinoma (determine its size and extent of metastases to lymph nodes and distant sites). In the absence of metastasis, treatment is likely to be surgery alone and a 5-year survival rate of 85% or better can be achieved. If the lesion were larger, implant radiotherapy might well be suggested. If the patient survives 10 years she is likely to be cured. However, 10% of oral carcinoma patients develop a second primary lesion in the mouth or upper aerodigestive tract. The chances of developing a second lesion are assumed to be reduced by stopping smoking and the patient should be encouraged to do so. Smoking-associated cardiovascular disease, if severe, may also compromise treatment.

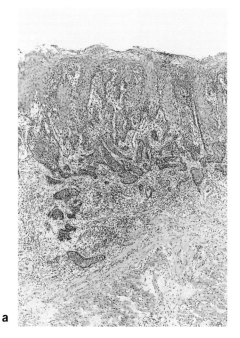
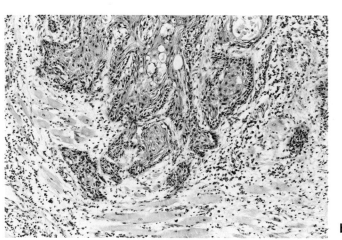

Fig. 31.2 The histological appearances of the lesion. **a** Lower power view; **b** higher power view.

Summary

A 30-year-old man is referred to your dental hospital by his general practitioner with a painful swelling of the right side of the face. What is the cause and what treatment would you provide?

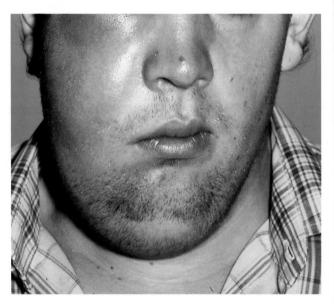

Fig. 32.1 The patient on presentation.

HISTORY

History of complaint

The patient has had toothache intermittently for many months. A few weeks ago the pain became excruciating and did not respond to analgesics. Then, suddenly, it reduced in severity and the patient thought it had resolved.

However, about 10 days ago a different pain developed. A tooth on the upper right has become very tender and he has not been able to bite on it. The swelling suddenly enlarged yesterday.

Over the last few months the patient has been prescribed several courses of antibiotics and he finished a course of oral erythromycin 2 days ago.

Medical history

The patient is otherwise fit and well.

EXAMINATION

Extraoral examination

The patient is shown in Figure 32.1. The swelling is hot, tender and firm centrally but peripherally it is almost painless and softer. It extends from the nose to the anterior border of the masseter and the lower eyelid is very oedematous and contains blood pigment as if bruised.

The swelling is not pointing extraorally. There are palpable tender lymph nodes in the upper deep cervical chain.

Intraoral examination

The patient has slight limitation of opening which does not significantly hamper examination. The sulcus adjacent to the upper first molar and both premolars is tender and slightly reduced in depth by a firm swelling. The upper first and second premolars and first molar have large amalgam restorations. However the patient indicates clearly that the second premolar is the cause of the pain and this tooth is slightly mobile and raised in its socket. It is very tender on percussion and nonvital on testing with ethyl chloride. The first molar and first premolar appear vital.

INVESTIGATIONS

■ *Which additional investigation is critically important? Why?*

Taking the patient's temperature. This gives a good indication of the systemic effects of the infection and reflects the amount of pus in abscesses and/or the tendency of the infection to spread. The patient has a temperature of 37.2°C.

■ *Would you take a radiograph?*

In this case radiograph is not a useful investigation. Tests of vitality are much more likely to identify the causative tooth and, in any case, there appears to be no doubt about the diagnosis.

However there are good reasons why taking a radiograph may not help or even be counterproductive:
1. It takes up to 3 weeks for radiographic changes to develop after pulp necrosis.
2. The radiographic features may mislead if you attempt to use them to diagnose loss of vitality. When root apices are radiographed with the maxillary antrum superimposed, the normal periodontal ligament appears wider. This may be confused with early apical changes on infection.

Both these problems are appreciated in Figure 32.2, the periapical radiograph of this patient, which is completely normal.

DIAGNOSIS

■ *What do these findings tell you?*

The combination of inflammation, the non-vital tooth and adjacent probable abscess indicate an odontogenic soft tissue

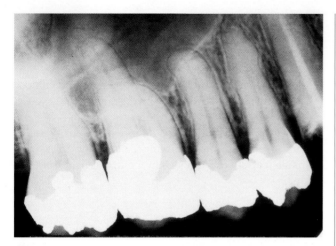

Fig. 32.2 Periapical radiograph showing the causative premolar.

Cause of swelling	Features
Oedema	Soft, not very red or hot, not tender on palpation and not painful. Compressible with slow continuous pressure. Often accounts for much of the facial swelling in children with odontogenic infection.
Abscess	Localized collection of pus which feels hard if small, tense or covered by a thick layer of tissues. If large it may be softer and exhibit fluctuance. Pointing to the skin or mucosa indicates abscess formation.
Cellulitis	Brawny, poorly localized swelling with marked tenderness and dusky redness. May contain small collections of pus but no large localized abscesses. Spreads, sometimes rapidly, through tissues. Usually associated with systemic symptoms, pyrexia, malaise, leucocytosis and lymphadenitis.

infection. The history of severe toothache which suddenly resolved suggests pulpitis subsequently relieved by necrosis of the pulp. The subsequent pain of a different character with a tender tooth suggests an apical abscess. The patient points clearly to the second premolar and this is almost certainly the cause of the pain because pain involving the periodontal ligament is well localized.

Trismus is an important sign, indicating that infection or inflammation has spread to involve muscles of mastication. However, trismus is not severe and probably results from inflammation and oedema of the buccinator and the anterior fibres of the masseter which lie at the posterior border of the swelling.

The infection has induced minimal systemic effects because the patient is not significantly pyrexic. Luckily, the infection appears to be localized. The firm centre to the swelling and the swelling in the sulcus will contain pus.

■ *What types of soft tissue infection arising from teeth cause facial swelling? How may they be distinguished and what is the relevance of doing so?*

Facial swelling may be the result of oedema, abscess formation, cellulitis or their combination.

It is important to determine which of these types of infection are present because the treatment and sequelae are different. Abscesses require drainage. Cellulitis requires aggressive treatment, usually including antibiotics, and oedema requires no direct treatment but resolves when the causative tooth is removed or the pulp treated.

Despite the fact that these terms are convenient, in practice most odontogenic soft tissue infections are caused by a mixed microbial flora and do not fall neatly into one category or another. It is not unusual to find an abscess with a surrounding zone of cellulitis and a degree of oedema is always present. Which type of infection develops is determined by the virulence of the pathogens (and synergy between species in the mixed flora), the resistance of the host and the anatomical constraints on the infection.

■ *If infections are not easily characterized, what are the important features on which treatment must be based?*

The critical factors which must be determined are whether:
● an abscess cavity is present (palpation, eliciting fluctuation);
● there is evidence of systemic effects (malaise, pyrexia, a toxic-shocked appearance);
● the infection is spreading rapidly (judged by the history and observation during treatment);
● the patient is predisposed to infection (from the medical history).

■ *Which type of infection is this?*

This appears to be primarily an abscess with surrounding oedema.

■ *In what tissue space(s) is the infection tracking/ localizing? What are the boundaries of this space?*

This abscess appears to be in the upper part of the buccal space. This is a potential space between the buccinator muscle and the facial muscles and parotid fascia, filled normally with loose connective tissue. Posteriorly it communicates with the masseter muscle and around the front of the ramus to the pterygoid space. Oedema spreads beyond the buccal space to involve the lower eyelid and anterior cheek in the canine fossa. The abscess is not yet pointing to the skin.

■ *Why has the infection localized here? Will it remain localized here?*

Abscesses arising from the canine, premolar and molar teeth which perforate the buccal plate of alveolar bone will spill out into the soft tissues either above or below the attachment of the buccinator. The attachment of the buccinator usually runs below the apices of the upper teeth so that infection is likely to pass superficially to the buccinator and into the cheek. If it passes below the attachment, an alveolar abscess or sinus will develop. Paths of spread of infection from an upper premolar are shown in Figure 32.3.

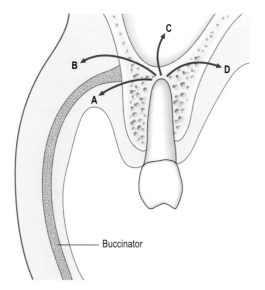

Fig. 32.3 Coronal section showing the paths of spread of infection from upper molars and premolars. Infection may pass buccally below the buccinator muscle into the sulcus or cheek intraorally (A), above the buccinator into the buccal space (B), into the sinus (C) or into the palate (D).

Despite being a thin muscle, the buccinator is a significant barrier to the spread of infection, which is unlikely to be able to perforate the muscle and develop a sinus into the mouth. Several sequelae are possible. Pus would be most likely to gravitate and spread through the whole buccal space down to the lower border of the mandible; it could point and then drain to the skin or spread laterally around the buccinator to involve other areas of the face, tissue around the masseter muscle or the pterygoid space. Its future course cannot be predicted.

■ *Is this a potentially life-threatening infection? If so, why?*

Not yet. Infection appears localized, the spread is not particularly rapid and there are no significant systemic symptoms. If a more spreading infection developed, the situation would change.

Involvement of the tissues around the eyelid is worrying. At present the swelling here is caused by oedema, but if infection were to spread to the upper lid or medial canthus of the eye the patient would be at risk of cavernous sinus thrombosis. This is a very rare but potentially fatal complication.

It would also be possible for the infection to spread posteriorly into the pterygomandibular space and infratemporal fossa. From here the infection could spread via veins to the cavernous sinus or middle cranial fossa.

■ *What is cavernous sinus thrombosis and what are its features?*

Thrombosis of the cavernous sinus follows spread of odontogenic infection along two main venous pathways. Bacteria and infected emboli travel posteriorly from the upper lip and face via the anterior facial vein. This connects via the ophthalmic veins to the cavernous sinus without valves to prevent retrograde flow. Alternatively, infection may spread from the pterygoid space via the pterygoid plexus of veins which connect directly to the cavernous sinus via the foramen ovale.

The local features are seen on one side at first but the signs become bilateral as the thrombus grows. The features are:

Local effects	Marked oedema of the eyelids
	Pulsating exophthalmos caused by venous obstruction
	A dilated facial vein
	Inhibition of movements of the eye
	Papilloedema and retinal haemorrhage
Systemic effects	Rapid pulse
	Marked pyrexia
	Severe malaise

In addition to treatment for the infection, thrombosis requires anticoagulation. The mortality rate is high.

TREATMENT

■ *What are the general principles of treatment for all odontogenic infections of the soft tissues?*

Treatment should be started rapidly. Infection may spread quickly and in some cases progress to a life-threatening situation with great rapidity. Identify patients with a risk of significant complications. Those at risk of airway obstruction, cavernous sinus thrombosis or showing toxaemia, suffering malaise or with a high temperature should be treated immediately, possibly even with parenteral antibiotics pending definitive diagnosis, and admitted to hospital for treatment.

Pus must be drained as soon as possible. With most infections causing swollen faces, effective drainage of pus and removal of the cause are the only treatment required. To ensure success, a drain may need to be placed in the incision.

Remove the cause as soon as possible. Removal of the causative tooth both prevents continuing infection and also drains the intraosseous abscess. The exception to this rule is when the cause is pericoronitis. In this case the soft tissue rather than the tooth is the cause and extraction can be detrimental (see case 21).

Provide antibiotic treatment if necessary. Antibiotics provide little benefit over drainage and removing the cause, but are often used and occasionally required. Pus should be collected on drainage and submitted to microbiology for culture and sensitivity investigation, in case a change of antibiotic is required subsequently.

Provide supportive measures. Ensure that the patient can eat, maintain a good fluid intake and rests. Consider admission to hospital until recovery has started and provide appropriate analgesia.

Review progress regularly. Daily review is appropriate for those treated on an outpatient basis. Those whose infection is serious enough to merit admission require more frequent review, between every hour and 6 hours depending on their status. If signs and symptoms do not improve progressively, further investigation and treatment is probably required.

■ *What are the principles of obtaining drainage? How will you drain the pus in this case?*

The principles of incision for drainage are:
- Take the anatomy into account and avoid incising near important structures.
- Incise only when pus has localized, unless rapidly increasing swelling is threatening the airway, in which case it should be drained as quickly as possible.
- Incise where the abscess is pointing or at the point of maximum fluctuation.
- Incise along the most direct route to the pus.
- If incision does not release pus, deepen the incision using blunt forceps, not a scalpel. Open the forceps blades to break open the abscess wall (Hilton's method).
- After incision explore, identify and open all locules of pus.
- Provide dependent drainage if possible.
- Place a drain if the abscess is large, deep or if the incision might close before the abscess resolves (for instance if the incision penetrates layers of muscle, fascia or skin which can move independently). Leave the drain in place for at least 12–24 hours, or until drainage stops.
- If possible, drain intraorally to prevent facial scarring and skin contraction.
- On the skin incise along Langer's lines or in a skin crease.
- On the skin, try to incise healthy skin. It will scar less.

In this case the pus lies between the buccinator muscle and skin. It is not pointing and is palpable in the upper buccal sulcus. Incision at this site under ethyl chloride spray anaesthesia is perfectly appropriate. However, the incision must extend through the buccinator to be effective, and some might prefer to obtain drainage with the patient under a short general anaesthetic.

■ *Should drainage ever be delayed?*

Occasionally drainage must be delayed until pus is properly localized into an abscess. If no pus can be identified on examination, incision will be futile. Waiting a day and providing antibiotics may induce pus to localize. Such a decision must be carefully considered.

■ *Will a drain be required?*

Quite probably. The abscess is not very deep but the incision must pass through a muscle. On the other hand, drainage will be dependent: the incision is being made below the pus and this will favour drainage. It may not be possible to decide in advance. If pus drains freely on incision and a cavity in the tissues is present, it would be sensible to place a drain, preferably a strip of corrugated rubber or, as a second choice, gauze. This should be sutured to the edge of the incision to prevent displacement. In this case a drain would be as easily placed under local as general anaesthetic.

■ *Can the tooth be conserved after soft tissue infection? How might you remove it?*

A soft tissue infection does not mean that the tooth has to be extracted and almost all could, in theory, be preserved. However, most such cases arise through neglect; the tooth is often badly broken down and is best extracted. Occasionally, when infection is spreading rapidly or if the airway is compromised the tooth is extracted to avoid delaying treatment, but even these severe complications do not require that the tooth be extracted. The critical factor is that drainage is obtained.

If the tooth is to be conserved, it must be opened and drainage effected through the pulp chamber in addition to draining pus by incision. Ideally the pulp chamber can be closed again fairly quickly. As soon as drainage ceases, the pulp chamber can be cleaned and a dressing placed. If pus continues to drain for some time, the chamber may be left open for up to 24 hours. After this period there is a risk that the oral flora may enter the tissues, reducing the chances of subsequent successful root treatment. Many clinicians will prescribe antibiotics because they consider drainage to be less effective when the tooth is retained.

Extraction is the more usual treatment. If local anaesthesia can be obtained and trismus is not severe, the tooth may be extracted at once. Infiltration anaesthesia is often difficult to achieve because of the low pH of inflamed tissues. Injection into infected tissue also carries the risk of spreading the bacteria more widely. Block anaesthesia is required.

A general anaesthetic may be necessary. If so, it will be convenient to admit the patient to hospital and complete all the surgical treatment at the same time. An anaesthetic may take some time to organize and in the meantime it would be appropriate to try to extract the tooth under local anaesthetic. A general anaesthetic should not be used in an attempt to overcome trismus. Forcing the jaws open will spread the infection.

If a surgical extraction is required, it may be delayed. As a general principle, surgery should be avoided if the surgical field is infected. However, this rather old rule is often not followed now, because of the availability of very effective antibiotic treatment. Some operators will perform a surgical extraction immediately, and the risk of spreading infection or inducing osteomyelitis seems to be extremely small.

In this case anaesthesia could not be obtained and so drainage and extraction were performed under a general anaesthetic. A short corrugated rubber drain was inserted.

■ *When should antibiotics be prescribed for odontogenic soft tissue infection?*

The attitude to antibiotic treatment varies between different centres. Antibiotics are unnecessary for the treatment of the majority of localized soft tissue abscesses and this is particularly so when pus collects superficially in the buccal sulcus or on the palate. Drainage and removal of the cause are much more important. However, in practice, many patients who require incision and drainage tend to be given antibiotics by clinicians, without a clear rationale.

Antibiotics should be prescribed if:
- The patient is prone to infection, for instance is diabetic or immunosuppressed.
- There is spreading infection (cellulitis).
- The airway is compromised.
- There is significant malaise, pyrexia or toxaemia.
- When the tooth is to be preserved rather than extracted. (The cause is not immediately eliminated.)
- Cavernous sinus thrombosis is possible.

Antibiotics prescribed for spreading infection may cause pus to localize, and drainage of abscesses may be possible a day or so later.

Antibiotics should never be provided as an alternative to draining pus.

What microorganisms cause odontogenic soft tissue infections?

Odontogenic soft tissue infections are mixed infections. The microbial flora usually contains about 25 species derived from the oral flora, of which about half are cultivable. Anaerobes outnumber aerobes by 10 or 100 to 1 and commonly isolated species are *Porphyromonas* sp., *Prevotella* sp., *Peptostreptococcus* sp. and *Fusobacterium* sp.; however, facultative anaerobes are usually present, often members of the *Streptococcus milleri* group. Although numerically a minor component of the flora, these organisms are important when selecting antibiotics.

If you decided to do so, which antibiotic would you prescribe initially? Explain why.

Almost all the organisms in odontogenic soft tissue infections are sensitive to penicillins. There is a small but increasing proportion of resistant strains but these do not seem to contraindicate penicillins. It is not necessary to prescribe penicillinase-resistant drugs just because one member of the microbial flora shows resistance and they are of no proven benefit in odontogenic infection. Penicillin V or G is sufficient provided drainage can be achieved.

Metronidazole is effective against the anaerobic species and is often prescribed. However, metronidazole should be used as an adjunct to a penicillin and never alone. It will kill the anaerobes but leave facultative anaerobes such as the *Strep. milleri* group unscathed. These organisms are capable of

causing a spreading soft tissue infection as a monoculture. Removing their anaerobic microbial competitors with metronidazole risks turning a relatively well localized mixed infection into a spreading streptococcal infection. In the wrong site this could be fatal.

In this case the patient received a single dose of 500 mg amoxycillin and 400 mg metronidazole intravenously during the anaesthetic. The same doses were prescribed orally three times a day for 5 days afterwards and this is an appropriate regime for most odontogenic soft tissue infections. However, as noted above, it may not have contributed greatly to the patient's recovery.

Why bother to take a specimen for culture and sensitivity testing?

As noted above, empirical treatment with penicillin with or without metronidazole is almost always effective. However, in some cases the infection stabilizes but fails to resolve. This may be due to inadequate drainage but a change of antibiotic may be considered a sensible precaution. The results of sensitivity testing may be helpful in selecting another antibiotic and identifying any unusual pathogens present. As culture and sensitivity testing takes about 3 days it must be requested as soon as a sample of pus can be obtained and before antibiotics are administered.

When interpreting the results of culture and sensitivity tests, it must be remembered that the organisms isolated are unlikely to be representative of the flora. Routine culture methods in most hospitals will detect only a few species, probably not the main component of the flora. Unless a change to a different antibiotic is clearly justified, it would be better to consider changing the dose and route of administration.

In order to be useful, the sample obtained for culture must be taken in such a way as to favour the growth of anaerobes and fastidious organisms. Ideally it should be taken directly from the abscess through a needle or through a sterile skin incision. Samples on swabs contaminated with oral flora are unlikely to be useful and may even provide a misleading result.

How quickly should the swelling resolve?

Patients may often feel much better within a few hours and a noticeable reduction in swelling, trismus, pain and pyrexia should be observed within 24 hours. By this time drains do not usually show pus and are removed and dressings placed over the site if extraoral. If there has been no resolution, the diagnosis, antibiotic treatment and effectiveness of drainage must be reviewed. Almost complete resolution should follow in 3–6 days, as in the present case.

CASE 33 Missing upper lateral incisors

Summary

A 15-year-old boy presents to you in general practice requesting closure of the spaces between his upper front teeth. What is the cause and how can a better appearance be achieved?

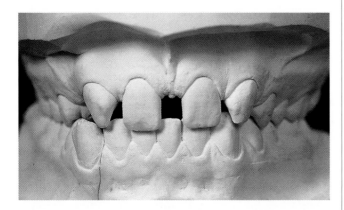

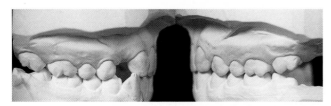

Fig. 33.1 Study models taken at presentation.

HISTORY

Complaint

The patient does not wish to have gaps between his upper front teeth.

History of complaint

His permanent teeth erupted at a normal age with large spaces between them. The deciduous predecessors had all been present and were exfoliated normally. None of the permanent teeth have been extracted.

Medical history

The patient is fit and well.

Family history

The patient's mother had a number of teeth missing. They had been replaced with a partial denture at an early age.

EXAMINATION

Extraoral examination

The patient has a skeletal class I appearance without facial asymmetry. There is a slight deviation of the mandible to the patient's left-hand side on opening, but no limitation of opening, temporomandibular joint clicks or crepitus or masticatory muscle tenderness.

Intraoral examination

The patient's soft tissues are healthy and his oral hygiene is good, with no calculus deposits, gingival inflammation or bleeding on probing. The teeth appear sound, with the exception of a buccal amalgam restoration in the lower left first molar.

Study models taken for treatment planning are shown in Figure 33.1.

■ *What features relevant to treatment do the study models show?*

Both upper lateral incisors are absent. From the front the upper central incisors are upright and separated by a large midline diastema. There is a mild class III incisor relationship, with a normal overjet but a reduced and complete overbite. The upper canines are mesially inclined and mesiolabially rotated, that on the left being more prominent. The lower right canine is labially placed, slightly distally inclined and in crossbite with the upper canine. There is mild lower labial crowding. The posterior teeth are well aligned and the first molars on the right-hand side are in a class I relationship and on the left-hand side in a half a unit class II relationship.

■ *What are the possible causes for the absent lateral incisors. What is the cause in this case?*

Missing	Developmentally absent, possibly associated with cleft lip or palate or other craniofacial syndrome
	Extracted
	Avulsed
Failure to erupt	Dilaceration and/or displacement as a result of trauma
	Scar tissue preventing eruption
	Supernumerary tooth preventing eruption
	Insufficient space as a result of crowding
	Pathological lesion (e.g. cyst or odontogenic tumour) preventing eruption

In this case the most likely cause for the missing lateral incisors is genetic absence. Genetic absence of some teeth is found in 3–7% of the population. The teeth most commonly missing are, in descending order of frequency, third molars, maxillary lateral incisors and second premolars. The absence of maxillary lateral incisors is a hereditary trait in about 1–2% of the population. The fact that the patient's mother wore a denture to replace missing teeth from an early age suggests a possible familial aetiology. Trauma or extraction and their related sequelae are readily excluded by questioning. The other causes are discussed in case 4.

INVESTIGATIONS

■ *What special investigations are required? Explain why for each.*

Investigation	Reason
Tests of vitality of the upper anterior teeth	To exclude incidental loss of vitality, to ensure that endodontic treatment is not required and that unsuspected loss of vitality does not compromise the subsequent treatment plan.
Radiographs	To determine whether the lateral incisors are present and unerupted and to exclude underlying lesions such as supernumerary teeth or cysts. Examination for this case should include a panoramic tomograph to provide a survey, exclude significant periodontal bone loss and confirm the presence or absence of third molars. In addition periapical views or an upper standard occlusal view are required for detailed analysis of the incisor region which suffers from superimposition in the panoramic view. Further films may be required to define the caries status.
The study models should be mounted on an articulator	To assess the occlusion and produce a diagnostic wax-up if required.

In this case all the upper anterior teeth responded to tests of vitality by ethyl chloride and an electric pulp tester.

■ *The panoramic tomograph is displayed in Figure 33.2. What does it show?*

The dental panoramic tomograph shows that the upper lateral incisors are missing with no evidence of supernumerary teeth or other lesions in this region. All other teeth were present including the unerupted third molars. This confirms the diagnosis that the upper lateral incisors are developmentally absent.

TREATMENT

■ *What are the main treatment options? What are their advantages and disadvantages?*

Option	Advantages and disadvantages
Space closure with adhesive restorations	Composite restorations added to the approximal surfaces of the central incisors and canines could reduce the spaces. This is the most conservative option, technically straightforward and might be acceptable as a provisional solution. However, complete closure could not be achieved with such wide diastemas and each tooth would look unacceptably wide.
Orthodontic space closure	This would bring the canine into the position of the lateral incisor requiring the shape of the canine to be modified by selective grinding of the tip and placement of composite to disguise it as a lateral incisor. However, the darker colour of the canine would be difficult to conceal, as would the gingival contour because of the canine eminence. The palatal cusp of the first premolar tooth is frequently visible and compromises the appearance. When the difficulty of complete space closure is taken into account, it is clear that this option is rarely ideal. It frequently produces a poor result despite being a time-consuming and costly procedure.
Create space for lateral incisors	Space creation by orthodontic treatment followed by provision of lateral incisors with a prosthesis involves a protracted phase of orthodontics and is costly. However it would produce the best appearance.

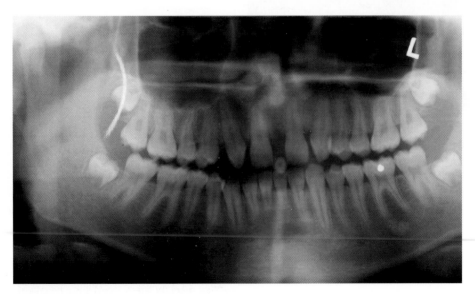

Fig. 33.2 Panoramic tomograph.

■ *The patient's main concern is his appearance. How would you demonstrate the possible results to him?*

The patient is considering committing himself to a long and complex treatment so the result of each of the treatment plans should be assessed with study models and diagnostic wax-ups. The possibility of the orthodontic treatment can be visualized by cutting the teeth off duplicate study models and fixing them in an orthodontically achievable position, the so-called Kessling set-up. Patient and dentist can then see what might be achieved by each treatment option.

Following discussion, the patient opts for the third treatment plan.

■ *How would you carry out the orthodontic treatment?*

The tooth movement demands fixed appliance treatment. Tooth tilting using a removable appliance would result in a poor appearance in the midline and produce spaces which are difficult to fill with a prosthetic replacement. If a fixed appliance is used the incisors may be more accurately positioned and derotation of the canines is possible. The orthodontic result for this patient can be seen in Figure 33.3.

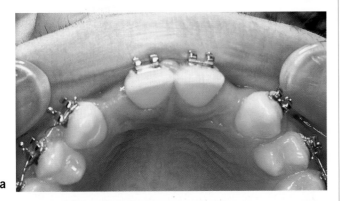

a

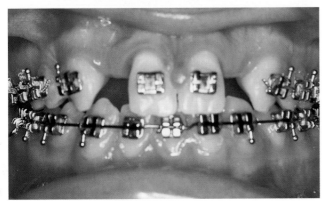

b

Fig. 33.3 The final orthodontic result.

■ *How would you now replace the missing lateral incisors?*

Prosthetic treatment should be as conservative as possible because the upper anterior teeth are vital and sound, and the patient is young. The teeth can be replaced with fixed or removable prostheses but the treatment of choice would be a minimum preparation bridge or bridges. Possible designs are shown in Figure 33.4.

Normally a fixed–fixed design in a minimum preparation bridge should be avoided. This is because debonding of one retainer will create an area of stagnation below it and risk caries. A typical minimum preparation bridge to replace a lateral incisor would be a cantilever design retained on the canine or central incisor.

However canine abutments (option A) would have a major disadvantage in this case. The canines were originally mesiolabially rotated and the orthodontic result is potentially unstable. Relapse would result in the pontics swinging out labially. An alternative might appear to be a cantilever design retained on a central incisor (option B) which has the

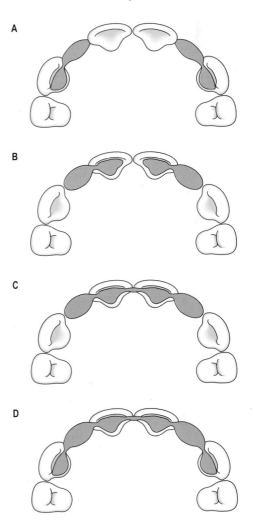

A

B

C

D

Fig. 33.4 Possible designs for minimum preparation bridge(s).

advantage of a greater enamel area for bonding. However, two separate cantilever bridges retained on the central incisors would also enable the orthodontic result to relapse and the midline diastema to reappear. Linking the central incisors together (option C) would prevent this but could not prevent the canines from relapsing to their original position.

A degree of orthodontic retention must be designed into the prosthesis and only a fixed–fixed bridge extending from canine to canine is suitable (option D). The potentially unstable orthodontic result may in itself favour debonding of one or more of the wings. Regular recall will be essential to detect this early. If debonding is a repeated problem, replacement with a conventional bridge may have to be considered. The need for orthodontic retention is the main reason that an implant retained solution is not appropriate.

The final bridge design and appearance are shown in Figure 33.5. Note how the orthodontic treatment plan must take into account the occlusal clearance required to cover the palatal surfaces of the canines.

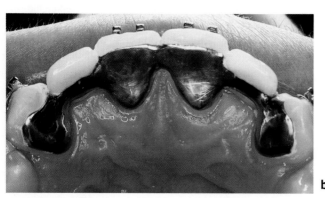

a

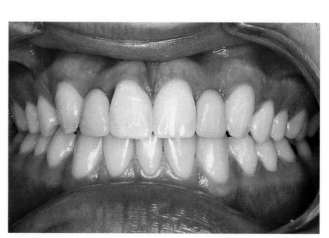

b

Fig. 33.5 The final result.

CASE
34 Anterior crossbite

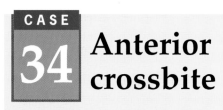

Summary

An 8-year-old girl is referred to you for an orthodontic opinion. She has an anterior crossbite. What is the cause and how would you treat it?

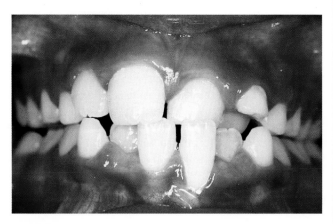

Fig. 34.1 The patient's appearance on presentation.

HISTORY

Complaint

The mother of the patient noticed the crossbite and is very anxious about her daughter's appearance. She requested a referral from the family's general dental practitioner.

History of complaint

The incisors erupted into their present positions and there is no history of trauma.

Medical history

The patient is fit and healthy.

EXAMINATION

Extraoral examination

There is no facial asymmetry and no clicks, locking or crepitus are present on examination of the temporomandibular joints.

Intraoral examination

■ *The appearance of the teeth on presentation is shown in Figure 34.1. What do you see?*

The patient is in the early mixed dentition stage and the teeth present are:

$$\frac{6\,E\,D\,C\,2\,1\,|\,1\,2\,B\,C\,D\,E\,6}{6\,E\,D\,C\,2\,1\,|\,1\,2\ \ \ \,C\,D\,E\,6}$$

The upper and lower incisors are crowded and the upper left central and lateral incisors are in crossbite. The lower left central incisor is labially placed and there is gingival recession and loss of attached gingiva to the mucogingival junction on its labial aspect. The oral hygiene is reasonable though mild interdental gingivitis is present around the poorly aligned incisors. The dental health is good.

■ *What specific features would you check in your examination? Explain why for each.*

See Table 34.1.

Table 34.1 Features to be examined

Feature	Reason
Can the patient achieve an edge-to-edge incisor relationship when closing on hinge axis?	On closing in a retruded position the patient makes initial contact on the lower left central incisor. If left untreated this could result in continued excessive occlusal loading on this tooth, causing further loss of support. The ability to achieve incisal contact is regarded as favourable because it indicates that minimal tooth movement should be required to correct the crossbite.
If so, is there an associated forward displacement of the mandible?	The initial contact on the central incisors displaces her mandible forwards into the intercuspal position shown in Figure 34.1. Early correction of the displacement activity may prevent possible temporomandibular joint dysfunction in later life. There is not yet significant wear faceting on the incisors. However, if they are left untreated, considerable attritional wear may develop.
How mobile is the lower left central incisor? Are probing depths increased?	Mobility is limited (grade 1) and probing depths are less than 2 mm. This would suggest that the prognosis for the tooth is good. If there were significant mobility or periodontal destruction extraction of the incisor might have to be considered as part of an orthodontic treatment plan.
How might space be provided to relieve the incisor crowding?	At the present stage of dental development, sufficient space would be provided by the extraction of deciduous teeth.

DIAGNOSIS

■ *What is your diagnosis?*

The diagnosis of crossbite has already been made by the patient's mother. The incisor crowding, gingival recession and anterior displacement of the mandible are the other significant factors requiring recognition.

■ *How would you assess the long-term prognosis for the lower left central incisor?*

At this early stage the recession may be reversible. The crossbite and premature contact are producing movement of the central incisor which is in danger of being pushed beyond the alveolus and losing its labial bone. The soft tissue defect is difficult to assess in the presence of slight inflammation. Some attached gingiva is almost certainly present labially and the recession seems to stop just short of the alveolar mucosal reflection. This patient has only a narrow band of attached gingiva as can be seen on the opposite side which is normal.

If the oral hygiene is improved and the crossbite corrected, the recession may also improve considerably. No additional attached gingiva will develop but further damage will be prevented. Further discussion of gingival recession around the lower anterior teeth will be found in case 3.

■ *What is the cause of the crossbite?*

Ectopic eruption of the upper incisors in association with crowding.

INVESTIGATIONS

■ *What special investigations would you require? Explain why.*

Radiographs are the most useful investigation for any orthodontic assessment. The following radiographic views are indicated:

View	Reason
Dental panoramic tomograph	As a general survey. Primarily to assess the presence or absence of permanent successors and any supernumerary teeth.
Upper standard occlusal	When considering active movement of the incisors, an upper standard occlusal may be useful in order to give more detail of the area around the incisor roots. When incisors are misaligned this view may reveal supernumerary teeth or odontomes or dilaceration as rare causes.
Periapical view	If you are concerned about the prognosis of the lower left central incisor a periapical film may help. This should be taken using a paralleling technique to assess bone loss. However, as noted in case 3, labial bone loss will not be visible in this view.

■ *The dental panoramic tomograph is shown in Figure 34.2. What does it show?*

The tomograph shows a normal dentition. The developmental age matches the patient's chronological age. All permanent successors are present and appear to be in favourable positions. There is not yet any evidence of third molar development, as is normal at this age. Though the panoramic view is not suitable for detailed diagnosis, there seems to be some mesial bone loss on the lower left central incisor.

TREATMENT

■ *What treatment plan would you propose?*

The incisor crossbite should be treated immediately to prevent further damage to the periodontium and attrition. Some authorities consider that early treatment will also reduce the possibility of temporomandibular joint pain dysfunction (myofascial pain) syndrome in later life. However, the evidence to support this contention is by no means conclusive.

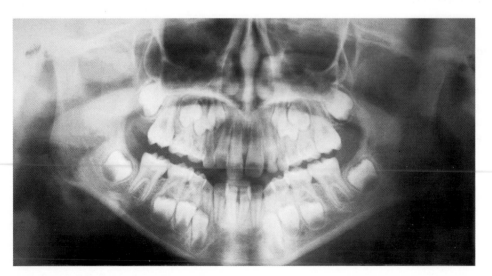

Fig. 34.2 Dental panoramic tomograph of the patient.

To provide space for relief of crowding and to allow the active tooth movements required to correct the crossbite, all deciduous canines and the deciduous upper left lateral incisor should be extracted.

An upper removable appliance is then fitted to correct the incisor crossbite.

■ *Design a suitable removable appliance to correct the crossbite.*

Only simple tilting tooth movements are required and these can be achieved most easily with a removable appliance. There would be no advantages to the use of a fixed appliance in such a case.

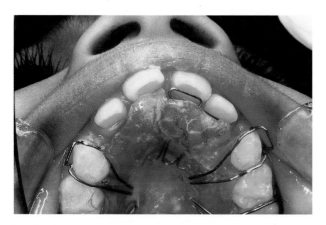

Fig. 34.3 The removable appliance used to correct the crossbite.

A suitable removable appliance is shown in Figure 34.3. It consists of:

• cribs on both upper Ds (0.6-mm wire)
• cribs on both upper first permanent molars (0.7-mm wire)
• T springs on the upper left central and lateral incisors (0.5-mm)

Treatment should take no more than 3–4 months as the amount of tooth movement required to correct the crossbite is minimal.

■ *Why is no posterior capping included on the appliance?*

Posterior capping would normally be considered beneficial when correcting a crossbite. Unless the teeth are held apart during treatment, the upper incisors cannot easily cross over the incisal edges of the lower incisors. Either an anterior bite plane or posterior capping would allow this.

In this particular case it was decided not to incorporate posterior capping as there is a reduced overbite and therefore minimal occlusal interference to the tooth movements. An anterior bite plane would not be indicated in such a case because eruption of the molars would further reduce or even eliminate the already small overbite.

■ *Figure 34.4 shows the patient at the end of active treatment. What do you see?*

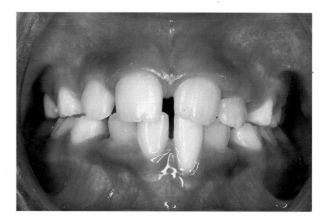

Fig. 34.4 The result after correction of the crossbite.

There has been an improvement in the incisor alignment and the crossbite has been eliminated. If you were able to examine the patient you would find that the mandibular displacement has disappeared.

The patient's oral hygiene has improved and the swollen rounded gingival contour seen in Figure 34.1 has resolved. There is still some slight gingival inflammation in the area of recession. It is difficult to judge whether there is a band of attached gingiva around the lower left central incisor. However, at this age the incisor is not fully erupted and enamel rather than root is exposed. The lower incisor has suffered premature gingival regression rather than recession. Follow up is required to check that sufficient attached gingiva remains until the patient is mature. It appears that no permanent damage has been suffered.

■ *What determines the stability of the orthodontic result?*

A positive overbite is necessary to maintain the corrected upper incisor positions in the short term. In the longer term, stability of the incisor position is dependent on the mandibular growth pattern which will determine the final overbite and overjet.

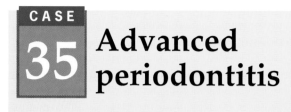

CASE 35

Advanced periodontitis

Summary

A 56-year-old man has severe periodontitis. Diagnose and plan treatment for his condition.

Complaint

The patient complains of loose back teeth, particularly the last tooth on the lower right.

History of complaint

He has recently moved to your area and has been a regular dental attender. His previous dental practitioner diagnosed periodontal disease several years ago and organized repeated courses of oral hygiene instruction and scaling. Despite this, several teeth are loose though he has suffered no pain.

Three years ago the remaining upper right molar teeth became very loose and were extracted when abscesses developed. Subsequently two implant fixtures were placed because he could not tolerate partial dentures. An implant-retained bridge was planned but the implants remain unused.

Medical history

The patient is fit and well and no illness was revealed by his medical history questionnaire.

■ *What questions will you ask the patient? Explain why.*

Ask about his tooth cleaning regime, because it is clearly failing. The patient tells you that he cleans his teeth three times a day using a modified Bass technique and changes his toothbrush at monthly intervals. He uses floss on his anterior teeth every day and occasionally on his molars and premolars where access is difficult.

Whether he smokes. Smoking is a risk factor for periodontitis.

Whether he is diabetic or has any other susceptibility to infection. This is relatively severe periodontitis and there is a history of multiple abscesses. These features do not

necessarily indicate an underlying condition but it would be worthwhile to exclude diabetes. Other features which might suggest diabetes are a period of rapid destruction in middle age, suggesting late-onset diabetes.

Extraoral examination

No cervical lymphadenopathy was present. The temporomandibular joint and mandibular movements appear normal.

Intraoral examination

The mucosa and soft tissues of the mouth were normal. The teeth present are:

$$\frac{4321 \mid 1234 \quad 78}{7654321 \mid 1234567}$$

Most molars contain small- to medium-sized amalgam restorations. No caries is detected.

The patient's oral hygiene is fair but the lower second molar teeth and upper left molars are mobile. The plaque control around the anterior teeth is good with minimal deposits of plaque or calculus. There is bleeding on probing around most posterior teeth and increased probing depths of 7–8 mm around the molars. No recession is present.

■ *How will you assess the patient's periodontal health and oral hygiene?*

They will be assessed by a combination of measurements and indices.

The measurements are:
- Recession
- Probing depths
- Attachment loss.

Recession and probing depth measurements are made at six points around the circumference of a tooth: mesially, at the midpoint and distally on the buccal and palatal surfaces. The distance from the cementoenamel junction to the gingival margin records the amount of recession. Probing depths are measured from the gingival margin to the base of the periodontal pocket. The sum of recession and probing depth gives the length of attachment loss.

The indices are described in Table 35.1.

The results of these examinations are shown in Figure 35.1. The lower right second molar is mobile to grade 3. All other molars are mobile to grade 2 and there is bleeding on probing from most pockets. The anterior teeth have only 2–3 mm probing depths and no bleeding on probing or gross attachment loss.

Table 35.1 Indices of oral health and periodontal hygiene

	Index score	Significance of score
Oral hygiene		Reflection of effectiveness of cleaning.
Degree 0	No plaque or debris	
Degree 1	Looks clean but material can be removed from the gingival third with a probe.	
Degree 2	Visible plaque	
Degree 3	Tooth surface covered with abundant plaque.	
Bleeding on probing		
Degree 0	None	Healthy or inactive disease.
Degree 1	Bleeding	Active disease. N.B. In smokers bleeding may be less than expected for the disease activity.
Tooth mobility		
Degree 1	Movement of the crown of the tooth between 0.2–1 mm in a horizontal direction.	Minor movement, possibly physiological. If periodontal disease present, treat conservatively.
Degree 2	Movement of the crown of the tooth exceeding 1 mm in a horizontal direction.	Caused by loss of attachment. The degree of mobility depends on remaining periodontal support and the shape of the roots. Conical roots on molars are more likely to develop mobility than divergent roots on teeth with a similar degree of attachment loss.
Degree 3	Movement of the crown of the tooth in a vertical and horizontal direction.	Indicates bone loss below the apex and little or no bony support. Usually indicates a need for extraction.
Furcation involvement		
Degree 1	Horizontal loss of supporting tissues not exceeding 1/3 of the width of the tooth.	Early furcation involvement, can be treated conservatively; predisposes to further and more rapid attachment loss if untreated. Much more difficult to keep clean.
Degree 2	Horizontal loss of supporting tissue exceeding 1/3 but not a 'through and through' lesion	Unlikely to respond to conservative treatment.
Degree 3	A 'through and through' lesion.	May be easier to clean depending on soft tissue contour. The prognosis for the tooth would depend upon the remaining amount of periodontal attachment and the length and shape of the roots. Indicates susceptibility to caries and risk of loss of vitality.

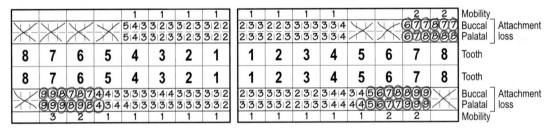

Fig. 35.1 The probing depths (in mm) at six points, bleeding sites (ringed) and mobility (grade), recorded for each tooth. No recession is present.

INVESTIGATIONS

■ *What further examinations or investigations would you perform?*

Vitality tests are indicated for all teeth with marked attachment loss or furcation involvement. This would include all molars.

■ *What radiographs would you take? Why?*

See Table 35.2.

■ *The dental panoramic tomograph is shown in Figure 35.2. What do you see?*

The panoramic film is of poor quality. The patient's head was not correctly positioned and this has produced a number of distortions. The lower border of the mandible appears bowed down and the lower anterior teeth are foreshortened. Spinal

shadows are also accentuated by poor positioning and the teeth in the midline appear out of focus because of superimposition. The head was also twisted, enlarging one side of the film. This can be seen most easily by looking at the molar crowns which are longer on the right than on the left. The patient's postoperative film in Figure 35.3 shows what the film should have looked like.

The radiograph shows extensive bone loss around the lower right and left second molars. The lower left second molar has bone loss and caries in the furcation. Furcation involvement was also evident on both lower first molars which were not as mobile.

■ *Where are the implants? How might you localize them more accurately?*

The panoramic view is insufficient to localize the implants accurately. They appear in focus but the focal trough in the

Table 35.2 Radiographic views

View	Advantages	Disadvantages
Dental panoramic tomograph (DPT)	This the appropriate initial view for periodontal assessment; also as a general survey for a new patient and to identify the number of implants present and their approximate site.	Distortion and poor resolution make detailed assessment of periodontal bone support and caries difficult, especially around incisors.
Full mouth periapical films	Ideal for assessing bone loss if taken with a paralleling technique. Selected films, based on the panoramic view, would be ideal and still involve a lower dose than full mouth films because the panoramic provides a dose equivalent to only 4 E-speed periapical films.	Not necessary: probing depths around the upper and lower anterior teeth were normal or only slightly increased. Full mouth films cannot be justified as an initial investigation on the basis of the radiation dose.
Vertical bitewings	Ideal for molars and premolars when there is no more than moderate bone loss.	The missing upper molars would have made the positioning of the films difficult, if not impossible.

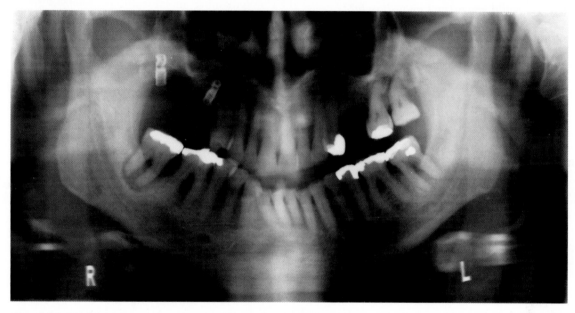

Fig. 35.2 Dental panoramic tomograph of the patient at presentation.

molar region is quite wide so that this gives no clue as to their buccolingual position. Their position and angulation will be critical in determining whether they can be used to support restorations.

If the end of the implant cannot be identified in the mouth, the implants could only be accurately localized using a tomographic technique, either CT scanning or multidirectional tomography. CT scanning is expensive and requires special software to prevent 'star artefact' shadows on the film. Multidirectional (spiral or epicycloid) tomography performed in machines such as the Scanora or Tomax produces cross-sectional images of any part of the jaws much more easily and would be the best method. If the implants were misplaced, the film might be taken with radiopaque markers on the ridge to aid localization. Alternatively it could be assumed that the implants are in an appropriate position and a flap could be raised.

■ *Are any other investigations necessary?*

Yes, a urine glucose test to exclude diabetes would be prudent. This was negative.

DIAGNOSIS

■ *What is your diagnosis?*

Chronic adult periodontitis, at a relatively advanced stage with considerable bone destruction around the molar teeth. There is grade 3 involvement of furcations on all lower molars and grade 2 involvement of the upper molars.

■ *This patient has problems with furcation involvement. What are the possible sequelae?*

- Devitalization of the tooth
- Further and more rapid periodontal destruction
- Periodontal abscess
- Root caries.

■ *This patient has already had courses of periodontal treatment. Why have they failed?*

Conservative periodontal treatment comprising oral hygiene instruction and scaling/root planing has been effective anteriorly. Posteriorly, where there are much deeper pockets and inaccessible furcations, further intervention is required to halt progression. Oral hygiene must improve around the posterior teeth, particularly interdental cleaning. The patient is flossing too infrequently and in any case such wide interdental spaces are more effectively cleaned with tape, brush floss or minature bottle brushes.

TREATMENT

There is a need for immediate extraction of those teeth with a hopeless prognosis. A further period of improved cleaning and assessment is required before a definitive treatment plan can be made. There is root caries in one furcation and a caries prevention regime is also required.

■ *Which teeth would you extract immediately?*

Both lower second molars require extraction. The right molar has no bone support and is almost certainly non-vital. Bone loss around the mesial root is compromising the first molar. The left molar is less severely involved but has extensive caries in the furcation which renders the tooth unrestorable.

All the remaining molars have a poor prognosis and extraction must be considered. The upper molars have furcation involvement and the fused roots will make conservative treatment difficult. The lower first molars also have a poor prognosis and may require extraction later. However, all these molars are grade 2 mobile at maximum and are in occlusion and functional. They could be preserved in the short or medium term. The patient has shown some ability to control his disease around the anterior teeth and a definitive decision on extraction could be delayed until an attempt has been made to stabilize the periodontitis. If these extractions are carried out, the patient will either have to accept a premolar to premolar occlusion or a prosthesis.

The patient did not wish to lose more teeth than absolutely necessary and accepted a plan to retain a completely natural dentition for as long as possible. The remaining molars will be retained for the time being. There is a risk of excessive bone loss if abscesses develop or disease progresses. Close follow up will be required.

■ *In the long term, what are the broad treatment options?*

The broad options are presented in Table 35.3.

Table 35.3 Broad treatment options

Treatment plan	Advantages	Disadvantages
Lower arch		
Plan A. Extract all lower molar teeth and either leave or replace with an acrylic or cobalt–chrome-based partial denture.	Simple approach with minimal need to treat the periodontal disease.	Transition to artificial dentition will be difficult especially with free end saddles in the mandible. Initially, acrylic dentures would be indicated in both jaws which may predispose to further deterioration of the periodontal tissues.
Plan B. Extraction of all lower molar teeth, provisional denture, and replacement of the teeth with implant-supported fixed or removable prosthesis.	The prognosis of the implants would be good and would eliminate the need for dentures.	This is a costly procedure but probably the most effective way to retain a molar occlusion.
Plan C. Conservative management with surgical investigation of the first molar teeth.	The only choice if the teeth are to be kept. The first molars are usually relatively easily cleaned and the root morphology makes preservation possible.	There is a cost implication of surgery and follow-up treatment, and the procedure is uncomfortable. Oral hygiene must be excellent to embark on this course of action.
Upper arch		
Plan D. Retain the upper left molars and treat conservatively. Leave the implants buried for future use.	Retains natural dentition, inexpensive. Retains natural occlusion for lower first molar. If these teeth can be retained, no prosthesis will be necessary.	Accepting teeth with a poor prognosis means that dentures or bridges must be designed with their future loss in mind.
Plan E. Extract molars. Leave the implants buried, accepting the existing premolar-to-premolar occlusion.	A simple and inexpensive procedure.	The implants would not be used. The discomfort and expense associated with their placement would be needless.
Plan F. Extract molars. Use the implant to retain a removable partial denture replacing all the missing teeth.	The restoration would be relatively simple and have good retention and stability.	An expensive route because of the need for precision attachments within the denture. Often the attachments in the denture wear and need replacement.
Plan G. Extract molars. Maintain the edentulous space on the left side and replace the missing teeth on the right with an implant-supported bridge.	The implants would be used to retain a bridge. Eating would be easier and teeth provided on one side.	The loss of teeth on the contralateral side may become a problem. The position of the implants may mean that a bridge is not suitable.

■ **What is the appropriate solution for this patient?**

This will depend largely on the patient who has expressed a wish to retain a natural dentition for as long as possible making plans C and D preferable. Some recommendations can be made:

- The implants should be retained for use later. These have been placed at some expense and provide an insurance policy for the future. If a molar occlusion can be retained, they are not required in the short term.
- A premolar-to-premolar occlusion provides acceptable function, though the appearance may be unacceptable depending on the visibility of the molar spaces.
- The upper molars provide useful occlusion and, though compromised, will probably last many years with conservative treatment. If the upper molars are to be retained, the lower first molar should be preserved if at all possible.
- Preservation of the lower right first molar would provide occlusion against the upper second premolar and possibly against an implant-supported prosthesis in the longer term. However complex treatment may be required and saving it might be regarded as a less essential element of treatment. The main reason for preserving it is that all the left molars may eventually be lost and it opposes the implants.

- Conservative treatment will take a long time and its success will depend primarily on the patient's ability to clean the teeth.

■ **What are the treatment options for the lower first molars? Under what circumstances are these possible and practical?**

See Table 35.4.

The patient quickly develops a more effective cleaning regime and root planing is performed. Over a period of 3 months the bleeding is eliminated and the mobility of all posterior teeth improves. There is still slight bleeding from the furcations of the lower first molars but the gingival condition is good. Conservative management appears to have been successful and more complex treatment options can be considered.

The following treatment is provided and the results are shown in Figure 35.3. Root resection is performed on the lower left molar and hemisection on the right. This eliminates the furcation and enables cleaning. The inflammation around the roots resolves.

Table 35.4 Treatment options for the lower first molars

	Treatment	Indications and contraindications
Eliminate tooth	Extraction	Very mobile; poor oral hygiene or compliance; patient wishes; caries in furcation or elsewhere rendering tooth unrestorable; insufficient bone support on either root to conserve. This option has already been discussed and rejected.
Retain furcation	Root planing alone	Effective only for grade 1 involvement. Inappropriate in this case where furcations cannot be debrided without raising a flap.
	Root planing with surgery	Still difficult; possible for lower first molars only. The chances of success are improved if the furcation contour is changed ('furcoplasty').
	Tunnel prep/apically repositioned flaps	Opens furcation for cleaning but also risks caries.
Eliminate furcation	Hemisection or root resection	Difficult procedure; expensive; hemisected tooth loses contact on one side; full coverage restoration may be required. Only suitable for teeth with bone far enough below the furcation to allow surgical access.

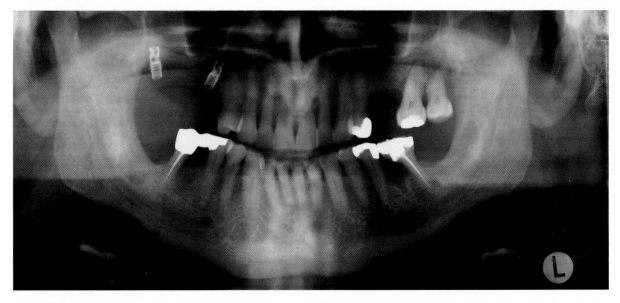

Fig. 35.3 Dental panoramic tomograph showing the result of treatment.

■ *Do the hemisected or root-resected teeth require restoration?*

Ideally, yes. The large area of exposed dentine and risk of fracture of the overhanging crown after root resection really demand full coverage restorations. However, complex and expensive treatment is often avoided because hemisected and root-resected teeth are compromised.

However, hemisected or root-resected teeth which have proved themselves stable over a period of months or years are best restored. In this case the hemisected molar root was linked to the premolar with a fixed movable bridge. Care must be taken that the design of the bridge does not overload the periodontal support of the root. Both teeth remain in function and are excellent semi-permanent solutions to this patient's problem.

Restoration, root treatment and surgery add up to a huge investment in time and money spent on one very compromised tooth root. If a definite need for a bridge or denture had been identified at the outset, an implant would have provided the support required at lower cost and with a better long-term prognosis.

■ *How do you assess the potential usefulness of the implants?*

The position of the implants is not favourable. Even on the panoramic view it can be seen that the fixtures are not parallel making them unsuitable for a fixed prosthesis. The fixtures are small, of different types and partially integrated. The mesial implant would appear to have less bone supporting it, and it is unclear whether it could support significant occlusal load.

CASE 36
A lump in the palate

Summary

A 32-year-old lady is referred to your hospital oral and maxillofacial surgery department by her general dental practitioner because of a swelling in her palate. What is the cause and what treatment is appropriate?

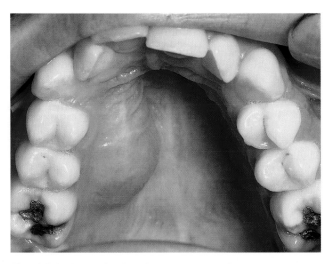

Fig. 36.1 The patient's palate on presentation

HISTORY

Complaint

The patient has noticed a lump but has experienced no pain.

History of complaint

The patient thinks that the lump has been present for at least a year, possibly two. It has enlarged slowly and is now starting to be a nuisance.

Medical history

Her medical history reveals no illness. She has recently given up smoking but previously smoked two or three cigarettes a day.

EXAMINATION

Extraoral examination

She is a fit and well-looking woman. No cervical lymph nodes are palpable and the temporomandibular joints appear normal. There is no facial asymmetry.

Intraoral examination

The appearance of the palate is shown in Figure 36.1. There is a swelling of the right side of the palate and maxillary alveolus. There is no caries and only a few relatively small amalgam restorations.

■ *What are the features of the swelling?*

The swelling has the following characteristics:

Site	Molar to central incisor region
Size	2 × 3 cm approximately
Shape	Oval
Surface	No ulceration
Colour	Overlying mucosa normal. Has a slight blue tinge
	No evidence of inflammation, not pointing
Contour	Regular, rounded

If you were able to palpate the lesion and the patient's neck you would discover the following:

Lesion consistency	Firm, not fluctuant
Lesion mobility	Fixed
Cervical lymph nodes	No submandibular or cervical lymph nodes palpable

DIFFERENTIAL DIAGNOSIS

■ *On the basis of what you know so far, what types of lesion would you include in your differential diagnosis?*

1. Benign neoplasm of palatal salivary gland, most probably a pleomorphic adenoma
2. Malignant salivary tumour, and if so:
   — most probably a mucoepidermoid carcinoma, *or*
   — polymorphous low grade adenocarcinoma,
   — but *possibly* an adenoid cystic carcinoma
3. Odontogenic causes:
   — *either* an abscess
   — *or* an odontogenic cyst, probably a radicular cyst
4. Mucous retention cyst
5. Antral or nasal lesion bulging into the mouth, for instance a carcinoma.
6. Miscellaneous other possibilities.

■ *Which of these possibilities are the most likely? Explain why.*

Benign salivary gland neoplasm. The site of the swelling is compatible with a palatal salivary gland origin though it is slightly more anterior than is typical. Salivary glands are more numerous in the posterior hard palate or soft palate and a swelling level with or behind the molars would be more characteristic of a salivary gland origin. If the lesion is arising in a gland, then a neoplasm is the most likely cause of a long-standing painless swelling. About half of minor gland neoplasms are benign and half malignant. By far the commonest single benign tumour is the pleomorphic adenoma and this is a very likely cause. Pleomorphic adenomas are commonest in middle and old age but have a wide age distribution and the young age of the patient need not exclude this possibility.

Malignant salivary gland neoplasms are equally common in minor glands, as noted above. If the tumour is malignant, then a mucoepidermoid carcinoma or polymorphous low grade adenocarcinoma would be the most likely causes because they are the most prevalent. Adenoid cystic carcinoma is rarer, but a very significant possibility because it requires more extensive surgery and carries a poor prognosis. The lack of ulceration and young age favour a benign neoplasm over a malignant one, but a malignant tumour is a definite possibility.

Dental causes must be considered because they are so common. The site would be very typical for an abscess arising from a nonvital lateral incisor or the palatal root of an upper first molar, but there are no symptoms or signs of acute infection. The slow and painless growth might suggest a cyst as a likely cause. However, the swelling appears to arise in the palate rather than the alveolus which is not expanded. Dental causes seem less likely than salivary gland causes, but as they are common it would be prudent to exclude them.

■ *Which of these possibilities are unlikely? Explain why.*

A mucous retention cyst is the most likely non-neoplastic salivary gland cause and the bluish tinge to the lesion suggests a cyst. However, this lump is firm and appears to be of long duration. A mucous retention cyst would be expected to burst or fluctuate in size if present over a long period. This lesion is rather large for a mucocoele on the palate.

Antral or nasal causes must be borne in mind but are also unlikely. Any lesion which had eroded through the palate or sinus wall would be expected to be ulcerated or inflamed.

INVESTIGATIONS

■ *What investigations would you perform?*

Tests of tooth vitality of all the teeth in the upper right quadrant are required to exclude the possibility that a non-vital

tooth is present and the cause of an abscess or cyst. Radiographs are required for these and other reasons.

■ *Which radiographic view(s) would you select? Explain why.*

A selection from the radiographic views shown in Table 36.1 is indicated for the reasons given.

The panoramic tomograph revealed no abnormality in the right palate or alveolus.

■ *Is a biopsy appropriate? What types of biopsy might be used and what are their advantages and disadvantages for this case?*

Yes. Only a biopsy will provide the definitive diagnosis. However, deciding whether or not to biopsy a salivary gland swelling is not always a simple choice. Inappropriate biopsy could do the patient a disservice. There are a number of possibilities, as presented in Table 36.2.

Either an incisional biopsy or FNA should be performed, and the choice will depend on the availability of cytology services in the clinic and the surgeon's preference.

■ *A fine-needle aspiration of the lesion was performed and the appearances of the aspirate are shown in Figure 36.2. What do you see?*

The cells are stained with the Papanicolaou stain which stains nuclei blue and cytoplasm green, or orange if keratinized. Figure 36.2a shows a sheet of uniform cells with moderate amounts of cytoplasm. Their cytoplasm, polygonal shape and cohesive growth indicate that these are epithelial cells and their uniform nuclei suggest they are benign. The second field, shown in Figure 36.2b, shows smaller numbers of spindle cells without significant cytoplasm in a matrix. Taken together, these appearances are characteristic of pleomorphic adenoma.

DIAGNOSIS

The diagnosis is pleomorphic adenoma.

Table 36.1 Selection of appropriate radiographic views

View	Reason
Intraoral views of alveolus	To exclude odontogenic or bony causes.
Oblique occlusal	To see whether the lesion has perforated or resorbed the underlying palate.
Panoramic tomograph or occipitomental view	To detect changes in the maxillary sinus if there were symptoms of sinus involvement.
Panoramic tomograph	General survey of jaws. The panoramic is not ideal for this lesion because it lies outside the focal trough of the tomograph.
Computerized axial tomograph (CT scan)	The palate cannot be visualized well by standard views and you might consider this as an initial investigation. It will give an excellent view of palatal erosion or perforation if present. However, it does entail a significant X-ray dose, waiting time and expense. A plain film would be a more appropriate initial investigation unless palatal perforation is suspected clinically.

Table 36.2 Possible biopsy types

Biopsy type	Advantages and disadvantages
Fine-needle aspiration cytology (FNA/FNAC)	Quick and accurate in most cases though a minority of such lesions will not be amenable to diagnosis by cytology. Nevertheless, usually accurate enough to give the definitive diagnosis and can be performed in conjunction with other biopsy types if necessary. Result usually available in 1 day.
Trucut or wide-needle biopsy	These provide a small tissue sample. Wide-needle biopsy is now little used because FNA is easier and more accurate. There is a risk of damaging important structures, though this is more of a problem in the parotid gland than in the palate.
Incisional biopsy	As a general rule, incisional biopsy risks spreading salivary neoplasms into the tissues. Pleomorphic adenomas, the commonest benign neoplasms, are often mucinous in texture and can spread into the fascial planes of the neck and up to the skull base or down to the mediastinum when incised for biopsy. However, this is more of a problem in submandibular or parotid glands. In these sites incisional biopsy should not be performed unless the lesion is thought to be malignant. Only then will the diagnosis influence treatment. In the present lesion, spread is not a particular concern. The top of the lesion is accessible and the entire biopsy site could be excised during definitive surgery if the lesion turns out to be malignant. There is no risk of spread to tissue spaces. An incisional biopsy could be performed.
Excisional biopsy	If the lesion were smaller then an excisional biopsy might be considered appropriate. A small margin of normal tissue could be excised on the assumption that the lesion is a pleomorphic adenoma. This would not be ideal. FNA or incisional biopsy are readily performed and it would be better to determine whether the lesion is benign or malignant before excision, to ensure that an appropriate margin is taken.

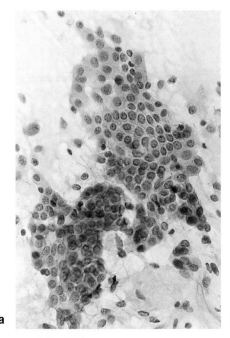 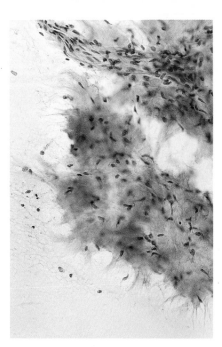

a   b

Fig. 36.2 a, b The appearances of the smear of cells taken by fine-needle aspiration.

TREATMENT

■ *How should this lesion be treated?*

The appropriate treatment is excision with a small margin, at least a few millimetres. The pleomorphic adenoma is benign but often incompletely encapsulated and simple enucleation often results in recurrence. The defect could be closed with either a temporary acrylic plate or local surgical flaps depending on the surgeon's preference. Radiotherapy is ineffective as a primary treatment, though it is sometimes used for widespread recurrences at other sites.

■ *Would you like further investigations before carrying out treatment?*

Although the pleomorphic adenoma is benign it can resorb bone by pressure. Before excising the lesion it is important to know whether the palate has been perforated because any postsurgical oronasal or oroantral fistula would have to be repaired. This lesion is relatively small and this step might be omitted, but with a larger tumour it would be an appropriate reason for carrying out a CT scan.

■ *The histological appearances of the excision specimen are shown in Figure 36.3. What do you see?*

Very different appearances are seen in different areas of the tumour (it is *pleomorphic*). Figure 36.3a shows sheets of epithelial cells in which there are small ducts containing eosinophilic material. At the edges of the sheets, cells separate and progressively merge with more dispersed cells in a myxoid stroma. These sheets and dispersed cells are the same cell types as those seen in the smear made from the fine-needle aspirate shown in Figure 36.2. Here they are seen in section, in their correct relationship to each other, whereas the smear is of whole cells spread onto a glass slide, hence their different morphology.

Figure 36.3b shows numerous small duct-like clusters of cells separated by a hyaline fibrous stroma. Many of the ducts have a bilayered structure with a partial outer layer of cells with clear cytoplasm.

Other fields shown incomplete encapsulation but a well demarcated periphery. These features are typical and diagnostic of pleomorphic adenoma. If the lesion appears excised histologically, cure is expected.

PROGNOSIS

■ *Are there any significant complications of pleomorphic adenoma? Are you concerned for this patient?*

Yes, carcinoma may arise in a long-standing pleomorphic adenoma and these *carcinomas ex pleomorphic adenoma* carry a very poor prognosis. However, this process takes many years, usually 10 or more, and is therefore seen mostly in elderly patients. This is an unlikely risk in this young patient with a short history. There is nothing in the history or examination to suggest malignancy and fine-needle aspiration, biopsy or examination of the excised specimen have excluded it.

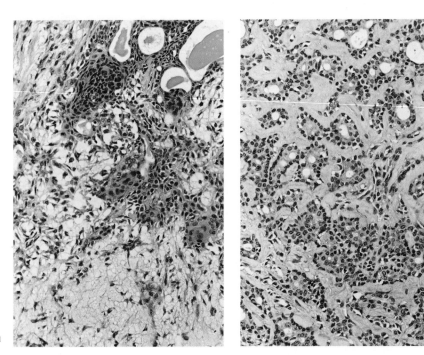

Fig. 36.3 a, b The histological appearances of the excision specimen.

CASE 37

Rapid breakdown of first permanent molars

Summary

A 7-year-old boy presents with first permanent molar teeth which his parents say have decayed rapidly, starting immediately on eruption. Identify the cause and discuss the treatment options.

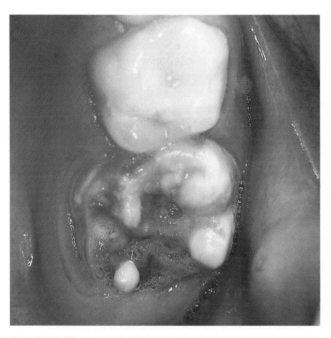

Fig. 37.1 The upper left first permanent molar.

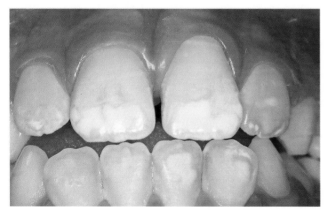

Fig. 37.2 The central incisors.

Complaint

The child complains of pain from his back teeth on both sides. The pain is worse with sweet foods and cold liquids and persists for several minutes after stimuli. Tooth brushing with cold water is also painful but the teeth do not cause pain on biting.

History of complaint

The pain has been present for a few months and has increased in severity over the last month. The child now reports that one of his back teeth feels broken. The first permanent molars erupted on time and his mother noticed that some of them appeared to crumble as soon as they emerged through the gum. She has read in magazines that fluoride can damage teeth and has switched to a toothpaste without fluoride on the assumption that this is the cause.

Medical history

The patient is a healthy child, the only history of note being neonatal jaundice.

Dental history

The child has no experience of operative dental care. A diet history reveals a reasonably well balanced diet, with limited consumption of refined carbohydrates and carbonated beverages. Toothbrushing has been performed with adult-formula fluoride-containing toothpaste, starting at approximately 1 year and continuing until 7 years of age.

Extraoral examination

The child has no facial swelling or asymmetry and no lymph nodes are palpable.

Intraoral examination

He is in the early mixed dentition stage. All four first permanent molars have areas of brown, rough, irregular coronal enamel. The severity varies between the teeth and the worst affected are the maxillary molars whose enamel appears to be completely absent in some areas. These teeth have soft dentine exposed occlusally. The lower right first permanent molar is the least severely affected with only a small localized brown enamel defect on the buccal aspect. This is hard on probing. In addition, there are areas of white enamel opacity in the incisal third of the labial surface of all permanent central and lateral incisors, which are most pronounced in the maxillary central incisors. The remaining deciduous dentition is caries-free, and appears normal in structure and morphology. Oral hygiene appears good. The appearances of the dentition are shown in Figures 37.1 and 37.2.

■ *On the basis of what you know already, what do you suspect?*

The defects appear to be hypoplasia of the enamel which has either become carious or taken up extrinsic stains. The molars are so severely affected that diagnosis is difficult, but the opaque white zones on the central incisors are characteristic of enamel hypoplasia. This term is often used loosely to include enamel hypoplasia (in which less enamel is formed) and enamel hypocalcification (in which the enamel is not fully mineralized).

■ *Do the enamel defects follow a chronological pattern, and if so, at what time was the affected enamel formed?*

Yes, the incisal and occlusal parts of the permanent central incisors and first molars form at about the same time, starting to mineralize just before birth. The affected enamel would have been formed after birth and during the first 1–2 years of life. This may be seen by consulting Figure 37.3.

■ *What additional questions would you ask, and why?*

The chronological pattern suggests systemic illness which may be identifiable in the history. Defining a possible cause may allow others such as fluorosis to be excluded. You need to ask further details about the prenatal and perinatal medical history. The following conditions may be relevant and should be specifically sought:
• Preterm birth or low birthweight baby
• Rhesus incompatibility
• Intubation as neonate
• Maternal vitamin D deficiency.
   These disturbances may manifest as enamel defects distributed along the enamel formed around birth. You should also enquire about all severe systemic disturbances in the first 2 years of life, for example meningitis, encephalitis, severe measles or pneumonia.

DIFFERENTIAL DIAGNOSIS

■ *What is the likely cause of the child's pain?*

The hot and cold sensitivity is characteristic of pain mediated by a vital pulp. It could be a result of caries in the dentine or exposed occlusal dentine.

■ *What is your initial differential diagnosis for the enamel hypoplasia?*

Dental caries is the commonest cause of destruction of first permanent molars and should be considered, even though the appearances would be very unusual. Enamel hypoplasia is more likely and developmental and acquired forms and/or generalized and localized forms are recognized. The most likely cause is enamel hypoplasia due to neonatal illness. Other causes which might be considered are amelogenesis imperfecta, fluorosis and cytotoxic chemotherapy for malignant disease. In some cases no cause is found and the term idiopathic enamel hypoplasia is used.

■ *Justify this differential diagnosis.*

Dental caries is the commonest cause of destruction of the dental hard tissues. Newly erupted teeth are particularly prone to dental caries until their enamel maturation is completed in the oral environment. First permanent molars are also prone to early caries because of their deep fissures. However the possibility of caries seems unlikely. Although there is no guarantee that the diet history elicited is truly representative of the child's actual diet, there are no restorations or caries in the deciduous dentition. The molars have discoloured or absent enamel over a wide area. This is not typical of dental caries unless carbohydrate intake is excessive or the teeth have some other predisposing factor such as enamel hypoplasia. The soft dentine indicates that some caries is present but the pattern of destruction suggests that this caries is secondary. The zones of opacity on the incisors look like early 'white spot' demineralization but are at a site which is almost never affected by caries.

Enamel hypomineralization and/or hypoplasia is the most common developmental disorder observed in teeth. This child has a generalized defect with a chronological pattern. The history of neonatal jaundice deserves some consideration. It is capable of affecting amelogenesis but rarely causes clinically evident hypoplasia and then only in very severely affected individuals. Neonatal jaundice is a very

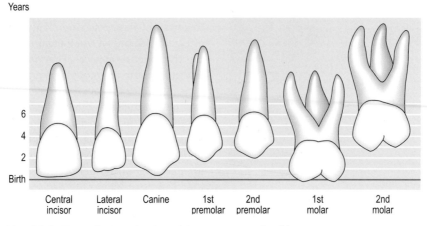

Years

Central incisor   Lateral incisor   Canine   1st premolar   2nd premolar   1st molar   2nd molar

Fig. 37.3 Time of mineralization of the permanent dentition.

common condition and in almost all cases can be excluded as a cause of enamel hypoplasia. In this child the position of the enamel defects is inconsistent with a short period of jaundice at birth.

Fluorosis where it is endemic, is a common cause of enamel opacities and enamel hypoplasia. The deciduous dentition is usually much more mildly affected. The level of fluoride required to cause enamel defects depends on concentration, period and age of ingestion.

Fluorosis is almost certainly not the cause of the current problem. The defects in the molars would result from only very high fluoride concentrations, in excess of 25 parts per million (p.p.m.). Such levels do not occur in the UK. In addition, fluorosis of this severity is endemic and should not follow a chronological pattern.

Mild fluorosis may be seen as a result of supplementation and this is presumably what the parent has read. In such cases there are usually fine opaque white lines following the perikymata and small irregular enamel opacities or flecks with or without staining. Such mild defects are also common in normal teeth and increase in frequency when the fluoride level is lower than 0.7 p.p.m. Although the severity of the defects and distribution are incompatible with the diagnosis of fluorosis, it needs to be considered because the child has been using adult-formula fluoride-containing toothpaste from an early age. Ingestion of adult-formula fluoride toothpaste would be the most likely cause of fluorosis. Fluoride toothpastes should not be used by children until they can rinse and spit out, at about the age of 7 years.

Amelogenesis imperfecta must be considered even though it is rare. Amelogenesis imperfecta can cause enamel hypoplasia, hypocalcification or hypomaturation and either of the first two conditions could lead to the appearances seen in the molar teeth. However several factors suggest that this is not amelogenesis imperfecta. There appears to be no family history, the pattern appears chronological rather than affecting all surfaces of all teeth equally and the deciduous dentition is unaffected. While these features are not conclusive because of the wide range of clinical presentations seen in the many different types of this disease, they do make the diagnosis most unlikely.

Idiopathic enamel hypoplasia is a convenient term used to describe cases of enamel hypoplasia for which no cause can be ascertained.

INVESTIGATIONS

■ *What investigations are indicated and why?*

Intraoral radiographs are indicated to assess the proximity of the coronal defects to the dental pulp. A panoramic tomograph is indicated, to ascertain the presence and stage of development of the remaining permanent dentition, in view of the possibly poor long-term prognosis of some of the first permanent molars. The panoramic tomograph is shown in Figure 37.4.

If there were extensive softening of the occlusal dentine of the molars or if radiographs indicated deep caries, tests of vitality would be required.

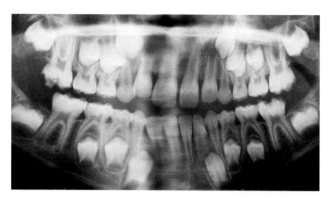

Fig. 37.4 Panoramic tomograph.

■ *What does the panoramic tomograph show?*

All permanent teeth with the exception of the third permanent molars are present and the dental age is consistent with the patient's chronological age. The gross structural defect in the first permanent molars is reflected in their radiographic appearance. The worst affected teeth – the maxillary molars – have irregular enamel outlines and there is reactionary dentine in the distal pulp-horns. The view is unsuitable for detailed examination of the teeth, but no large carious lesions are evident and the unerupted permanent second molars appear to be of normal shape and to have a normal enamel structure.

DIAGNOSIS

■ *What is your diagnosis?*

The patient has enamel hypoplasia in a chronological pattern, and in the absence of a known insult to account for the defects; idiopathic enamel hypoplasia/hypomineralization is a reasonable working diagnosis. The diagnosis may need to be reviewed if evidence of early illness can be obtained from the general medical practitioner or if more teeth erupt with similar defects. The diagnosis is sufficiently accurate to embark on treatment.

TREATMENT

■ *What treatment options are available for the molars?*

The appropriate treatment for grossly hypoplastic first permanent molar teeth is extraction, particularly when, as here, caries is also present. Preservation of these molars through adulthood would require provision of full-coverage crowns. These have a finite lifespan and their intermittent replacement, the risks of undetected leakage, caries and pulpal involvement, localized periodontitis and the expense and inconvenience would amount to significant morbidity in the lifetime of the patient.

■ *When should the molar teeth be extracted?*

Timing of the extractions is important and several factors must be taken into consideration:

Factor	Reason
Stage of dental development	Second permanent molars are most likely to erupt passively into a favourable position when there is radiographic evidence of calcification of a small crescent of interradicular dentine (mineralizing of the furcation). This is the ideal time to extract the first molar and is generally between $8\frac{1}{2}$ and $10\frac{1}{2}$ years of age.
Presence of third molars	This must be assessed radiographically. Hard tissue formation should be visible at age 9–10 years. The follicle may be visible as early as 7 years.
Orthodontic analysis	A complete assessment must be made. The space gained might be utilized for active orthodontic treatment. Extraction of first permanent molars is rarely ideal for orthodontic purposes and treatment may be complex. If no third molars are present, the need for orthodontic treatment may be critical in deciding whether or not to extract the first molars.

■ *How can the molar teeth be preserved until the patient is at the optimal age for their extraction?*

Preformed stainless steel crowns are a durable, cheap and relatively simple restoration. Laboratory-made nickel–chrome onlays have been advocated as a less destructive option, should it be decided that the teeth are to be retained for full coronal coverage restorations in later life. A preventive resin restoration can be provided for the less severely affected molar in the lower right quadrant.

■ *What treatment options are available for the incisor teeth?*

The areas of white enamel on the labial surface of the incisor teeth do not require treatment at this age and they may become less obvious with time. Should an interim cosmetic improvement be required in the patient's teenage years, composite veneers applied by hand, with no tooth preparation,

provide a simple and effective solution. The advantages and disadvantages of the possible restorative solutions are listed in Table 37.1.

■ *What advice would you give the mother with regard to fluoride?*

The misconception about fluorosis should be dispelled: fluorosis can only develop while the teeth are forming. Provided the child can rinse and spit out effectively it would be appropriate for him to use an adult-formulation fluoride toothpaste. This would provide a significant caries benefit (and the mother would also gain from using it). No fluoride supplement is indicated for this child who, at least on the basis of a preliminary analysis, eats little sugar and has no caries. There would be a particular advantage in using fluoride toothpaste during adolescence and early adulthood when the diet often changes markedly.

Table 37.1 Possible restorative options for the incisors

Technique	Advantages	Disadvantages
Composite veneers	Not destructive of tooth tissue, reversible and generally well tolerated even in anxious children. Excellent cosmetic result possible and easy to maintain.	Discolour with time. Tendency to fracture if placed at incisal edge.
Enamel microabrasion	Minimal destruction of enamel if carefully performed. Technique well tolerated.	Unpredictable. Teeth may suffer postoperative sensitivity. Accidental exposure of dentine is possible where enamel is very thin.
Localized composite restoration	Enamel destruction limited to defect and full thickness need not be removed if opaque composites used. Good cosmetic result possible.	Irreversible, weakens tooth structure and large areas of dentine may be uncovered. Colour change and marginal discolouration with time.
Porcelain veneers	Good appearance	Contraindicated in this age group as gingival contour not mature and stable tooth position not yet established.
Full crown restoration	Good appearance	Inappropriate until late second decade because immature pulp horns may be exposed. Gingival contour not mature and stable tooth position not yet established.

CASE 38

A complicated extraction

Summary

A 35-year-old man attends your general dental practice surgery requesting extraction of a tooth.

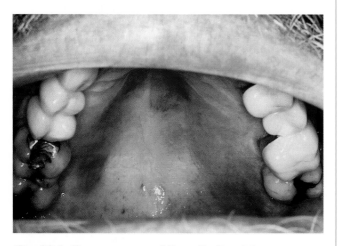

Fig. 38.1 The appearance of the patient's palate.

HISTORY

Complaint

He points to the lower left second premolar and says that the tooth is very tender to touch.

History of complaint

The tooth has been tender for some months and root canal treatment at another surgery was initially successful but has proved ineffective in the longer term.

Medical history

The patient's medical questionnaire indicates no relevant medical conditions.

EXAMINATION

Extraoral examination

The extraoral examination is normal except for a few palpable but normal-sized lymph nodes in his right and left cervical chain.

Intraoral examination

You immediately notice that the patient's oral mucosa is not normal. The appearance of the palate is shown in Figure 38.1.

The lower left second premolar has a large amalgam restoration and is tender to percussion. A sinus is present over the apex and the tooth does not respond to a test for vitality.

■ **What do you see in the patient's mouth?**

- The palate appears bruised with two purple-coloured lesions, one on each side of the palate extending from the gingival margin up the sides of the vault. Neither lesion appears to be raised above the surface.
- There is a discrete sharply defined slightly red patch in the anterior palate, just to the left of the midline.
- There are a few scattered red spots on the soft palate.

■ **What do these changes tell you?**

Individually none of these lesions can be diagnosed on the basis of the appearance alone. However in combination the appearances are almost diagnostic. The purple lesions appear vascular and could be haemangiomas or another blood vessel lesion including Kaposi sarcomas. The red patch has the characteristic appearance of erythematous/chronic atrophic candidiasis. Both lesions are associated with immunosuppression, and you should immediately suspect HIV infection because Kaposi sarcoma is extremely rare with other causes of immunosuppression. In this clinical setting the palpable lymph nodes also support this diagnosis. It is almost certain that the patient is HIV-positive.

■ **What do you need to know? What would you say to the patient?**

You need to identify whether the patient is aware of his HIV infection but has chosen not to tell you the full medical history, or whether he is completely unaware of it. Almost all patients who know that they are HIV-positive will tell their dentist provided they are asked in an appropriate manner. Sometimes patients withhold the information because of previous insensitive management, a dentist having refused to provide treatment or because they are worried that practice confidentiality cannot be relied on. However, your questions need to be phrased to take account of the fact that the patient may be unaware of his HIV infection. It is very important that you approach this matter with sensitivity. You could adopt the following line of questioning.

- Tell the patient that he has some unusual signs in his mouth which you cannot easily explain. Ask whether he has noticed them.
- These changes may be infections. Enquire whether he knows of any reason why he might be particularly prone to infection.
- Point out that there are several possible reasons for being prone to infection and that it would be worthwhile investigating further to find the cause. Proffer examples such as anaemia, immunosuppression as a result of steroid therapy or viral infection. Patients who know that they are at risk of HIV infection may often use the prompt of a viral infection to discuss the possibility.
- If the patient indicates that they are HIV-positive, ask whether you might have their clinic address so that if

necessary you may make contact for medical advice relating to dental treatment.

- If the patient gives no indication that they are HIV-positive, they should be referred to their general medical practitioner or to a specialist oral medicine or oral surgery unit for further investigation.

It is inappropriate to ask questions about lifestyle or sexuality. Even pointing out that HIV infection is one potential cause of the oral signs may not be well received in a dental setting. It would be reasonable to check the medical history questionnaire, including whether the patient has recorded coming into contact with someone with HIV infection or AIDS.

If the patient discloses HIV infection you should respond positively and acknowledge that you will respect the confidentiality of this sensitive information.

■ *What other oral signs may be associated with HIV infection?*

Diseases strongly associated with HIV infection

Candidiasis

    Erythematous

    Pseudomembranous

Hairy leukoplakia

Periodontal disease

    Linear gingival erythema

    Necrotizing ulcerative gingivitis

    Necrotizing ulcerative periodontitis

Kaposi's sarcoma

Lymphoma

Lesions less commonly associated with HIV infection

Mycobacterial infections

Melanotic pigmentation

Necrotizing (ulcerative) stomatitis

Cystic salivary gland disease

Thrombocytopenic purpura

Nonspecific ulceration

Viral infections including *Herpes simplex*, *Herpes zoster* and human papilloma virus infection.

In addition a wide variety of unusual infections may be found more rarely.

■ *Which of these signs are specific for HIV infection?*

None. All may be seen in other types of immunosuppression and many can be found in normal patients, albeit very rarely.

DIAGNOSIS

The patient readily informs you that he is HIV-positive and has only recently been diagnosed. He is aware of the Kaposi sarcomas which were the presenting sign of HIV infection. He has just started on combination drug therapy.

The lower left second premolar has a periapical abscess draining via a sinus.

TREATMENT

Extraction of the tooth is indicated.

■ *Is it appropriate that the tooth should be taken out in a general practice surgery?*

The General Dental Council advocate that patients with HIV should be treated in general practice. Denying this patient treatment on the grounds of having HIV infection alone would put you in breach of the GDC and BDA guidelines and might lay you open to a legal case under the Disability Discrimination Act 1995.

However, when a patient has late or symptomatic HIV infection, their medical history may become so complicated that a referral to a specialist dental clinic is appropriate. Referral may not be possible in an emergency situation and treatment, including extractions, may need to be carried out in a general practice setting.

■ *You will need medical advice. How will you obtain it?*

People with HIV usually attend outpatient hospital clinics and the patient's general medical practitioner may not have the most up-to-date test results. These clinics are usually extremely helpful if telephoned for information. However the patient's right to confidentiality must be respected at all times. Firstly, the patient's permission must be obtained to telephone and secondly, it is enough to explain to the clinic what you propose to do and to request the results without mentioning the patient's disease status or irrelevant information.

■ *What additional information would you require from the patient's HIV management clinic? Why?*

See Table 38.1.

CD4 T lymphocyte counts and the viral load, a measure of HIV viral RNA in the blood, are often known to the patient or may be given by the clinic. These indicate the level of immunosuppression and infectivity, respectively, but are not directly helpful in predicting whether a patient is likely to bleed or be at risk of infection after an extraction.

■ *Should the tooth be taken out without this extra information?*

No, in a general practice situation that would be unwise.

■ *Would any special infection control precautions be required for the extraction?*

No, the patient should be treated normally. It is assumed that all patients have the potential to carry an infectious disease and dental practices should have one level of infection control ('universal precautions') for all patients. (However it should be

Table 38.1 Further information needed from HIV clinic

Information	Reason
Is the patient prone to infections?	Antibiotics may be prescribed in immunosuppression when they would not normally be considered necessary, but should be reserved for patients with known susceptibility to infections. This is because the risk of adverse effects such as candidiasis and diarrhoea resulting from disturbance of the normal flora is increased in HIV infection.
Neutrophil count	Patients may be neutropenic. Neutrophils provide the first line of defence against infection and if the circulating count is less than $1-1.5 \times 10^9/l$, postoperative antibiotics may be appropriate.
Platelet count	Bone marrow suppression in late HIV infection causes thrombocytopaenia. The normal number of platelets is $150-400 \times 10^9/l$, but they do not usually fall to a low enough level to cause bleeding problems until late disease. However, this patient has signs of late disease (Kaposi sarcoma) and the red spots on the palate are probably petechial haemorrhages.
Does the patient have co-infection with hepatitis B or C?	These infections are not uncommon in HIV-positive individuals. Liver damage may cause a coagulation defect that could complicate the extraction. It also disturbs drug metabolism.
The names of the drugs that he is taking	Some of the retroviral drugs have significant interactions with other classes of drugs (see below). The patient is taking zidovudine (AZT), zalcitabine (ddC) and indinavir.

noted that additional precautions may need to be taken for patients at risk of, or suspected of suffering from, a transmissible spongiform encephalopathy such as Creutzfeldt-Jacob disease (CJD) and new-variant CJD.

■ *What antiretroviral treatment might the patient be taking?*

There are three classes of antiretroviral drugs, each with several members:

Protease inhibitors	Zidovudine (AZT)
	Didanosine (ddI)
	Zalcitabine (ddc)
	Lamivudine (3TC)
	Stavudine (D4T)
Nucleoside reverse transcriptase inhibitors	Saquinavir
	Indinavir
	Ritonavir
	Nelfinavir
	VX-478
Non-nucleoside reverse transcriptase inhibitors	Neverapine
	Delaviridine
	Loviride

■ *Do these drugs interact with any likely to be prescribed in general dental practice?*

Yes, and the interactions may be significant (Table 38.2). See also the notes on prescribing antibiotics in the table above on additional medical information.

■ *The clinic tells you that the patient has a platelet count of $45 \times 10^9/l$ and a neutrophil count of $1.9 \times 10^9/l$. There is no co-infection with viral hepatitis. Will you take out the tooth?*

No. The platelet count is too low. Bleeding problems would be expected if the count is below $50 \times 10^9/l$. You arrange with the clinic for the patient to be treated in a specialist centre.

■ *The patient asks to return to your practice for routine treatment. What is your reaction?*

Yes, he should be able to have routine dental treatment without problems though further extractions would require referral. Block analgesia is possible provided the platelet count remains above $30 \times 10^9/l$. Combination therapy is usually very effective and his oral signs will probably disappear in time and

Table 38.2 Interactions with antiretroviral drugs

Drug	Antiretroviral drug	Effect
Metronidazole	ddI, ddc, D4T	Additive toxicity. Increased serum levels of metronidazole.
Aminoglycosides	AZT, ddI, ddC, 3TC, D4T	Increased serum levels of the antiretroviral.
	Indinavir	Increased serum levels of the antiretroviral and additive toxicity.
	Ritonavir	Additive toxicity.
Corticosteroids	ddI, ddC	Additive toxicity.
Midazolam	Protease inhibitors	Increases serum levels of midazolam.
	Non-nucleoside reverse transcriptase inhibitors	Potential for interaction and increased or decreased serum levels of midazolam.
Lignocaine	Protease inhibitors	There is a theoretical risk of impaired lignocaine metabolism. The significance of this is unclear in the dental setting but it would be prudent to avoid approaching the accepted maximum dose.

platelets rise in number. Antiretroviral drugs may cause dry
mouth and this is a risk factor for caries. People with HIV are
also more prone to attachment loss with gingival recession.
However, standard preventive regimes should be effective
against any periodontal problems or caries that might develop.

CASE 39

Difficulty in opening the mouth

Summary

A 40-year-old Indian man presents to you in your general dental practice with limitation of mouth opening. You must identify the cause and institute appropriate follow up.

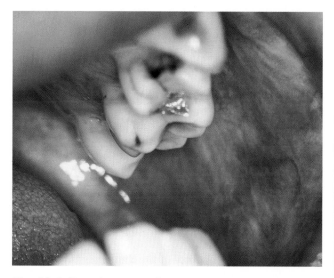

Fig. 39.1 Buccal mucosa, photographed at maximum mouth opening.

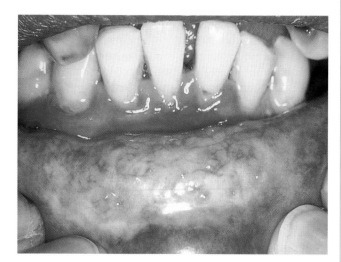

Fig. 39.2 The lower lip mucosa.

Complaint

The patient complains of difficulty in eating. He cannot open his mouth widely enough to place a proper mouthful of food inside and also has difficulty chewing.

History of complaint

He has noticed the reduction of his mouth opening over a period of several years but has never sought advice. It has not been painful though he has felt a burning sensation from his oral mucosa on eating during the same period. This varies in intensity.

Medical history

The patient is otherwise fit and well.

■ *What are the causes of limitation of mouth opening and how may they be classified?*

Limitation of opening is most frequently caused by trismus. By definition, trismus is caused by spasm of the muscles of mastication, though the term is often used loosely when opening is prevented by oedema or inflammation of the muscles or joint. Trismus is usually temporary.

Permanent limitation of opening may be caused by scarring of the soft tissues around the joint or mandible or by fusion of the condyle to the glenoid fossa (ankylosis). The causes may be divided as follows:

Trismus	Inflammation in and around the temporomandibular joint Trauma (fractures and/or soft tissue injury) Tetanus and tetany Temporomandibular joint (myofascial) pain dysfunction syndrome Soft tissue infection around the jaws or joint (usually dental in origin)
Permanent limitation of opening	A. *Extra-articular causes* Fibrosis due to burns or irradiation. Oral submucous fibrosis Mucosal scarring, e.g. in epidermolysis bullosa B. *Intra-articular causes* Congenital ankylosis Traumatic ankylosis Ankylosis following pyogenic arthritis Ankylosis following juvenile arthritis Neoplasms and other causes of enlargement of the condyle

■ *What questions would you ask?*

The patient should be asked whether there has been trauma or irradiation to the skull, temporomandibular joint or face and whether there have been any episodes of swelling of the face or around the joint. He should also be asked whether he uses betel quid (*pan* or *paan*).

The patient gives no history of trauma, irradiation, inflammation or infection. However, he has been a betel quid chewer for more than 20 years.

EXAMINATION

Extraoral examination

The patient looks mildly anaemic. There is no facial asymmetry or evidence of scars or inflammation around the joint. No tenderness can be elicited from the muscles of mastication. There are no clicks or crepitus or tenderness associated with the temporomandibular joint and no mandibular deviation on opening the mouth.

■ *What measurement would you take?*

The maximum voluntary mouth opening. The normal interincisal opening in an adult is approximately 30–40 mm. Measurement will provide a baseline reading against which to judge treatment or progression. It will also indicate the feasibility of dental and other intraoral treatment.

This patient can achieve an interincisal opening of 17 mm.

Intraoral examination

■ *The oral mucosa is shown in Figures 39.1 and 39.2. What do you see?*

The buccal and soft palate mucosae are paler than normal though some mucosal pigmentation consistent with the patient's skin colour makes this less obvious. When the mouth is opened fully, thin white hard bands run vertically just below the buccal mucosa. These are just visible in the picture and are much more readily felt as hard ridges. Some of the less pale areas are red and atrophic.

The same changes are found on the labial mucosa where bands of hard pale scar-like tissue are visible below the epithelium when the lip is everted. The gingival mucosa has lost its stippled appearance and there is oedema and rounding of the gingival contour consistent with gingivitis or periodontitis. There is some dark red/brown betel quid stain on the teeth.

If you were able to examine the patient you would find that he also has some reduction in mobility of the tongue and cannot protrude it very far. Most of the mucosa feels firm.

DIAGNOSIS

■ *What is your diagnosis?*

The presentation and features are characteristic of oral submucous fibrosis. There has been gradual limitation of mouth opening and restriction of tongue movements in a betel quid user who shows typical mucosal blanching and fibrosis as bands down the buccal mucosa. None of the alternative causes would produce these signs and symptoms.

■ *What other features of oral submucous fibrosis might be seen?*

In the early stages some patients complain of vesiculation of the mucosa. In severe cases with extensive tongue involvement the filiform papillae are lost.

■ *What is betel quid chewing?*

A habit practised by many people in the Indian subcontinent, much of south-east Asia and some parts of Africa. The basic quid comprises pieces or paste of areca nut and slaked lime, wrapped and tied into a packet in a vine leaf. A variety of other components is usually added; the combination varies between regions, but tobacco is almost always included together with flavouring agents such as cinnamon, cloves and ginger. The areca nut contains alkaloids which have a psychoactive effect and make the habit addictive. The quid is not chewed continuously but placed in the buccal sulcus and occasionally chewed. Many users have a quid in their mouth all day and some sleep with a quid. It has been estimated that 10% of the world's population use betel quid and chewing is a major health problem in many countries.

■ *What are the possible effects of betel quid chewing?*

- Oral submucous fibrosis
- Oral and pharyngeal squamous cell carcinoma
- Periodontitis, recession and root erosion at the site of use
- Tooth staining
- Decreased taste sensation
- Worsening of asthma
- Possible association with diabetes and other malignancies.

■ *What is the significance of the diagnosis? What else would you look for?*

Oral submucous fibrosis is a premalignant condition. Tobacco and other carcinogenic agents in the quid make quid chewing one of the highest known risk factors for oral carcinoma.

The patient's oral mucosa must be carefully examined for carcinoma and premalignant lesions. The features of early carcinoma and potentially malignant lesions are discussed in case 31. Approximately one-third of patients with submucous fibrosis have oral white patches and dysplasia is present in the mucosa of up to 16%. Malignant transformation to squamous cell carcinoma occurs in between 5% and 8% of cases.

The second significant feature is the restricted opening. This is often progressive and responds poorly to treatment. In the late stages of disease the patient may be unable to open the mouth at all and incisor extractions may be required to allow feeding. Limited opening is a major handicap for diagnosis and treatment of malignancy and premalignant lesions. It makes examination, detection and treatment extremely difficult and the prognosis for oral carcinoma in a patient with submucous fibrosis is very poor, mostly as a result of late diagnosis.

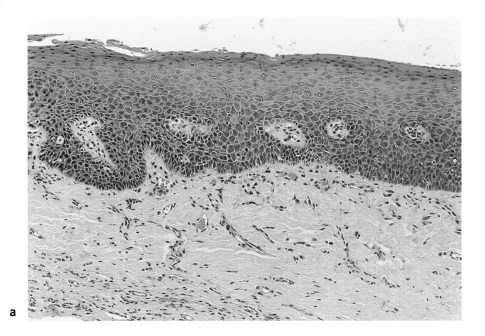

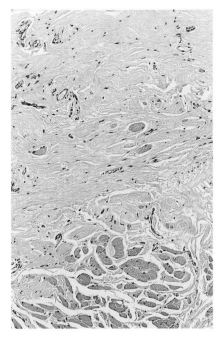

Fig. 39.3 Biopsy from the quid site: **a** buccal mucosa; **b** underlying tissue.

INVESTIGATIONS

■ *What investigations are required? Explain why.*

Biopsy is required to assess dysplasia. If there are lesions suspicious of malignancy, red or white patches or areas of otherwise abnormal mucosa they should be sampled for microscopy. More than one biopsy may be required. If no particular part of the mucosa is suspect, a sample should be taken from the area where the quid is held in the mouth.

The biopsy will probably also provide evidence to support the diagnosis of oral submucous fibrosis. However, in such a typical case biopsy for this purpose alone would not be justified. It might be considered in an early case where the diagnosis is in doubt.

■ *Would you perform this patient's biopsy in a general practice setting?*

No. This patient is at high risk of developing an oral carcinoma and the biopsy and further recall should be carried out in a specialist centre. Further discussion about when to biopsy potentially dysplastic mucosa will be found in case 31.

■ *A biopsy from the quid site is shown in Figure 39.3. What do you see and how do you interpret the findings?*

The mucosa is covered by epithelium which is atrophic and parakeratinized. The thickness of the normal buccal mucosa is about twice the thickness from the surface to the dermal papillae in this specimen. It is normally nonkeratinized except for a thin layer near the occlusal line. The epithelium is largely well organized and stratification and maturation are not particularly disordered; the epithelial layers are easily differentiated. There is an expanded basaloid cell layer comprising rather disorganized small and darkly staining cells which show anisonucleosis (nuclei of different sizes) and irregularly shaped, often angular, nuclei. Towards the centre of the epithelium there is a cluster of prickle cells between two dermal papillae showing early and single cell keratinization. These features amount to mild dysplasia. Below the epithelium there is even fibrosis of the connective tissue and scattered lymphocytes.

The deeper tissue shows the fibrosis of the connective tissue more prominently. All the tissue between the epithelium and underlying muscle is replaced by relatively acellular dense fibrous tissue. The superficial muscle is atrophic and is being replaced by fibrous tissue. Occasional residual muscle fibres lie in the fibrosis. This deeper tissue is uninflamed.

The fibrosis involving deep muscle is consistent with the diagnosis of submucous fibrosis and the overlying epithelium shows mild dysplasia.

Table 39.1 Treatment options

Option	Potential value
Habit intervention	Although areca nut is the main aetiological factor for oral submucous fibrosis, there are a number of other carcinogens. Therefore, cessation of the habit rather than altering the composition of the quid should be the aim. As a partial measure, discouraging tobacco in the quid would be valuable. This will reduce the chances of developing malignancy but limitation of opening may still worsen. Cessation is best but there would still be a risk of malignant transformation.
Regular review	The only reliable method for detecting dysplasia and early malignant transformation. Repeated biopsy may be required.
Muscle-stretching exercises	These appear to give good results in some patients. To be effective the muscle stretching must be frequent and prolonged. Bite wedges or a screw appliance may help produce the forcible opening required. Effective exercises are painful and patients must be highly motivated.
Intralesional steroids	These have been widely used, but the results are not encouraging in most patients and any benefit may not be maintained.
Surgical treatment	Occasionally used as a last resort. The fibrosis extends deeply into muscle and surgical excision of the scar tissue is rarely possible. Postoperative scarring replaces the original fibrosis and surgery is usually followed by relapse.
Nutritional supplementation	Many patients are deficient in iron and vitamins. Dietary supplementation with these and carotenes or vitamin A may be helpful in reducing progression but the effect is not marked.
Experimental methods	The lack of effective treatments has led to trials of many compounds, including interferon-gamma, but none has proved consistently useful.

TREATMENT

■ *What questions would you ask the patient about his betel quid habit?*

You need to know whether the patient includes tobacco in his quid, how many he uses each day and whether he sleeps with one in place. In addition you should check other smoking habits, because most quid users smoke as well, and some smoke traditional coarse unfiltered Indian cigarettes consisting of a rolled uncut tobacco leaf (*bidi* or *beedi*). Some users also practise a form of snuff dipping, placing ground quid constituents (*pan masala*) loose in the sulcus.

■ *What are the available treatments or treatment options? What is the potential value of each?*

See Table 39.1.

No treatment regime is satisfactory and the aim is maintenance and prevention of complications. If patients are committed to opening exercises, they may be spared the worst effects of limited opening. However, if disease is advanced at diagnosis, progressive limitation is likely. The best results are seen in those who have relatively localized disease at diagnosis, perhaps limited to the site of quid placement.

The aims are best achieved by helping the patient to cease the habit and by detecting malignancy or dysplasia as early as possible. If suspicious lesions develop they may be treated using the same modalities of treatment as in other patients, trismus allowing. All abnormal mucosa must be regarded with the utmost suspicion and a biopsy performed.

■ *What is the role of the general dental practitioner in such a case?*

Dental practitioners have an important role in the prevention of betel quid chewing just as in the prevention of smoking, primarily to prevent oral carcinoma rather than submucous fibrosis (a rarer effect of betel quid chewing). As noted above, most chewers also smoke and health workers need to address both tobacco habits.

The majority of those who regularly chew betel quid are from low socioeconomic groups and, at least in the UK, are often poorly informed of the health risks. Health education for chewers is most important and may need to be extended to other family members. The difficulty of convincing patients to give up should not be underestimated. The habit is addictive and is embedded in the cultural, social and religious customs of many ethnic groups. Many justify chewing on the basis of supposed health benefits which are accepted in their culture. The general practitioner can help the specialist centre to modify the risk behaviour, reinforcing the message to remove tobacco from the quid and encouraging patients to reduce the areca content and chew less frequently. The importance of prompt referral and regular mucosal examination for dysplastic lesions and carcinoma has already been stressed.

In the small number of patients who develop submucous fibrosis, dental treatment involves difficult choices and would be best carried out in a specialist centre. Initially treatment is not a problem and could be readily performed in general practice. However, some restorative treatment will be rendered impossible as restriction of opening progresses, and a thorough regime of effective preventive treatment must be adopted as soon as possible. Extraction of teeth with even small carious lesions or moderate periodontitis may become necessary, though it should be left until the last possible moment. It is still possible to restore and clean some teeth in late disease, though both activities are compromised. Every effort should be made to retain a stable occlusion to prevent progression to permanent overclosure.

CASE
40 Tooth wear

Summary

A 35-year-old policeman presents having noticed that his anterior teeth are becoming shorter. Identify the cause and outline options for management.

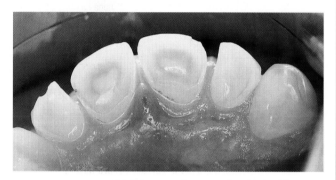

Fig. 40.1 Palatal view of the upper anterior teeth.

HISTORY

Complaint

The patient has become increasingly aware of his shortening front teeth. He is not greatly concerned about the appearance but feels that continued wear will eventually destroy the teeth completely.

History of complaint

He has noticed that his teeth have become worse over the last 3–5 years but cannot remember when he first noticed the signs. The patient has always attended a dentist regularly and has relatively few, small restorations and good oral hygiene.

Medical history

The patient is generally fit and well. He drinks about 10–20 units of alcohol each week.

EXAMINATION

Extraoral examination

The patient is a fit-looking man and slightly overweight. No submandibular or cervical lymph nodes are palpable. The temporomandibular joints appeared normal and there is no evidence of hypertrophy of the masseter muscles.

Intraoral examination

■ *The appearance of the anterior teeth is shown in Figure 40.1. What do you see?*

The palatal surfaces and incisal edges of the upper incisor teeth are worn. The wear involves the enamel and dentine but not the pulp. The palatal surfaces of the teeth appear smooth and unstained. The incisal edges are rough, small chips of unsupported labial enamel having fractured away.

If you were able to examine the patient, you would find that some of the upper and lower anterior teeth do not contact each other in the retruded contact and the intercuspal positions. All other teeth appear normal and the palatal surfaces of the upper posterior teeth are unaffected.

■ *What does this appearance signify?*

This is *tooth wear*, the loss of dental tissues through the processes of erosion, attrition and abrasion. Although each process may act alone, significant tooth wear is usually the result of a combination of these processes and erosion is often dominant.

The smooth surfaces suggest that erosion is a factor in this case and the distribution of enamel loss suggests that regurgitation of gastric acid may be the cause. Dietary acids are usually associated with erosion on the buccal or labial surfaces of the upper anterior teeth but if the patient rinses or swills acidic drinks in the palatal vault prior to swallowing, the pattern of erosion is very similar to that seen when gastric acid is regurgitated. Either source of acid might be the cause.

■ *Define erosion, abrasion and attrition.*

Erosion is the chemical dissolution of teeth by acids.

Attrition is the wear of tooth against tooth. Mild degrees of attrition are normal.

Abrasion is the wear of teeth by physical means other than the teeth.

DIFFERENTIAL DIAGNOSIS

■ *What is your differential diagnosis for this patient?*

1. Dental erosion caused by gastric acid combined with attrition.
2. Dental erosion caused by dietary acids combined with attrition.
3. Attrition alone.
4. Industrial erosion.

■ *Which of these causes would you exclude? Explain why.*

Attrition as a single factor is most unlikely to be the cause, because surfaces of the teeth do not contact in the intercuspal or retruded contact position. It would also be most unlikely that occlusal wear could affect the whole of the palatal surfaces of all incisors equally. Attrition is often associated with marked bruxism but there is no evidence of masseteric hypertrophy on examination.

Industrial erosion is now very uncommon. Acid present in the air of the working environment causes dental erosion but improvements in health and safety at work have almost eradicated this condition. Car battery acid workers used to suffer erosion, particularly affecting the buccal surfaces of the teeth. The patient's profession as policeman means he is unlikely to be exposed to an acidic environment though some patients may be exposed to volatile acids through hobby activities.

■ *What specific questions would you ask? Explain why.*

Tooth wear is often multifactorial and the patient must be questioned about all causes.

Do you suffer acid regurgitation from the stomach? Regurgitation of stomach acid can be noticed by the patient because of the taste. However, it may be unnoticed if it happens at night, and may or may not be associated with symptoms of gastric disease. Occasional mild reflux into the oesophagus or pharynx is relatively common.

What is your alcohol intake and what is the pattern of consumption? The patient has indicated an intake of 10–20 units of alcohol each week. Patients often under-represent their intake and it would be worth checking this with the patient. Many alcoholic drinks are acid, contributing to dietary acid (below), and binge patterns of drinking are often associated with vomiting. The possibility of a history of chronic alcoholism should be considered.

Do you have a high consumption of acidic foods or drinks? This is a common cause of dental erosion. The intake of both acid foods and drinks must be ascertained, together with the way in which they are consumed.

Do you grind or clench your teeth during the day or at night? Bruxism or other parafunctional habits are common causes of increased wear.

Have you ever suffered from an eating disorder such as anorexia or bulimia nervosa? These causes of gastric regurgitation need to be excluded. Such eating disorders are uncommon in males but their incidence is increasing.

In response to your questioning, the patient denies frequent acid intake, vomiting or bruxism. However, he indicates that he does suffer some acid regurgitation associated with his dyspepsia (heartburn) and that alcohol is sometimes associated with the attacks. He has had heartburn and regurgitation for 20 years but is not taking any regular medication to relieve the symptoms. He had not considered this significant enough to mention on his medical history questionnaire.

INVESTIGATIONS

■ *What investigations would you perform?*

A thorough dietary record should be taken by the patient to determine the true consumption of acidic foods and drinks. Diet analysis sheets need to be filled in for 4 or more days, including a weekend, and it is emphasized that the patient should write down all the foods and drinks taken over that time, including between-meal snacks. Both frequency and amount need to be noted and the patient should be specifically told to note suspect foods such as carbonated drinks, citrus fruits and drinks, vinegar and white wine, to ensure that none are missed.

Study casts of the patient's teeth should be taken. These will provide a baseline record against which progression of erosion can be detected. Tests of tooth vitality and intraoral radiographs might be taken if it is suspected that the wear has compromised the vitality of the pulp in any teeth.

Diet analysis confirms the patient's statement that he has a low consumption of acidic food and drink. This excludes dietary acid as a cause, leaving gastric acid as the only other source. Regurgitation erosion occurs when the stomach juice passes from the stomach into the mouth. The pH of stomach juice is around 1 or 2, and if regurgitation occurs frequently the damage to teeth can be catastrophic.

FURTHER DIFFERENTIAL DIAGNOSIS

■ *How might gastric acid enter the mouth?*

1. Gastro-oesophageal reflux disease
2. Eating disorders
3. Chronic alcoholism
4. Rumination.

■ *What features of these conditions might aid definitive diagnosis?*

Gastro-oesophageal reflux disease is usually associated with heartburn (intermittent retrosternal pain radiating along the oesophagus, worsened by lying down or a recent large meal), or epigastric pain (centred over the xiphisternum). When symptoms are related to meals, the term dyspepsia is sometimes used. In most patients symptoms of gastro-oesophageal reflux are self-limiting and little or no acid enters the mouth. In others complete regurgitation into the mouth is frequent, pain becomes persistent and patients seek medical advice. A small proportion of patients treat their pain with over-the-counter antacids and are unaware of the potential for damage to their teeth or oesophagus. A history of taking antacid preparations is a useful indicator for the activity of gastro-oesophageal reflux disease, and this patient has already indicated that he has noticed some regurgitation. This is the most likely cause.

Eating disorders are a cause of erosion in younger patients. Both anorexia nervosa and bulimia nervosa tend to affect young, adolescent, intelligent females with a history of overprotective parents. Anorexia is self-destructive. Sufferers lose body weight by starving themselves and/or vomiting to lose weight in an attempt to improve their body self-image. A small proportion of patients with severe anorexia die from the disorder. Unlike anorectics, bulimic patients usually have a stable body weight. They eat and drink in binges and vomit to control their body weight. There may be an accompanying history of drug and alcohol abuse.

Alcoholism. As noted above, alcoholism is associated with dental erosion, either through vomiting or the low pH of some alcoholic drinks.

Rumination is an unusual practice, being the habitual chewing of food, swallowing and then regurgitating it mixed with stomach acid to be chewed and swallowed again. It is considered rare but there is no accurate information on its prevalence and it is thought to affect young, healthy and mainly professional people. If the habit is continued it can cause significant damage to teeth.

The patient gives a clear history of regular heartburn and symptomatic regurgitation. He denies rumination and alcoholism and there is no suggestion of an eating disorder, an unlikely possibility in this age group.

DIAGNOSIS

■ *What is your diagnosis?*

The diagnosis is tooth wear caused primarily by erosion. The cause of the erosion is gastric acid reflux secondary to gastro-oesophageal reflux disease.

TREATMENT

■ *How will you manage the patient?*

The patient should be referred to a gastroenterologist or his general medical practitioner for further investigation of his symptoms. Reflux may be caused by a reduction in pressure around the lower oesophageal sphincter (as for instance in hiatus hernia) or abnormal oesophageal motility. Referral is necessary to detect such associated conditions and, if symptoms merit, to consider treatment with drugs which block acid secretion.

A conservative approach should be taken to treatment of the erosion. No immediate treatment is required if the erosion is relatively minor, as the patient is happy with the appearance of the teeth. If the cause is identified and treated, erosion will cease or progress more slowly. Study models taken at yearly intervals may be compared to those taken at the initial visit to assess progression, and if the tooth wear progresses, restorations may be considered.

In the early stages of erosion provisional plastic restorations will protect the palatal surfaces from further damage. However the short lifespan of such restorations commits the patient to further treatment. Alternatively palatal veneers of porcelain, composite or metal provide a longer term restoration if there is sufficient space occlusally for the restorations.

■ *What precautions must be taken to prevent iatrogenic damage when restoring worn teeth?*

Accurate diagnosis is essential. If attrition rather than erosion is diagnosed, occlusal splints might be prescribed. These would worsen erosion caused by gastric regurgitation because acid would be trapped beneath the splint away from the pH-neutralizing effect of saliva. There is also the potential for unglazed or unpolished porcelain to wear the enamel of the opposing teeth. This might become significant if there is an element of attrition causing the wear or if the restoration were allowed to occlude against dentine.

41 Worn front teeth

Summary

A 60-year-old man presents at your general dental practice saying that his teeth have worn down. What is the cause and how should he be managed?

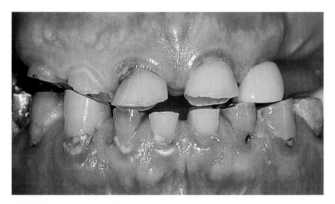

Fig. 41.1 The patient's appearance at presentation.

HISTORY

Complaint

The patient is unhappy about his short and discoloured upper anterior teeth. He is also finding that he has difficulty eating. The appearance of his teeth has recently become more important to him because he has taken a job in which he deals with the public. He wishes primarily to improve his appearance and appears to be sufficiently motivated to complete a course of complex dental treatment.

History of complaint

The patient has only recently started to attend his dentist regularly, after a 10-year period without treatment. Most of his posterior teeth were extracted before the age of 45 and he has worn his present upper partial denture for at least 12 years.

EXAMINATION

Extraoral examination

No submandibular or cervical lymph nodes are palpable, the temporomandibular joints appear normal and there is no tenderness around the muscles of mastication. Despite the anterior tooth wear there is no evidence of loss of occlusal vertical dimension.

Intraoral examination

The oral mucosa is healthy. In the mandible all teeth between the left and right second premolars are present but in the maxilla there are only five anterior teeth remaining. The appearances are shown in Figure 41.1.

Wear of the incisal edges of upper and lower anterior teeth has produced short clinical crowns and the upper right lateral incisor and canine are worn almost to gingival level. There are deposits of plaque around the cervical margins of his teeth and a number of teeth have cervical caries. Despite the plaque, there is only occasional interdental bleeding on probing and no significant increase in pocket depths. The upper ridges are not extensively resorbed and are broad and well defined. When asked to bite his teeth together the patient adopts the forward mandibular posture shown in Figure 41.1.

Both lower lateral incisors and the lower left canine and first premolar appear discoloured. Only the lower left second premolar fails to respond to an electronic test of vitality.

The patient produces his acrylic upper partial denture from his pocket. It is poorly retentive and of indifferent fit.

■ *What is your differential diagnosis? What features suggest each possibility?*

The patient is suffering tooth wear. This is usually caused by a combination of three basic underlying processes: erosion, attrition and abrasion. In this case it seems likely that the cause is predominantly erosion with attrition as a secondary factor.

Aetiological factor	Features
Erosion	Erosion is usually caused by excessive dietary acid or regurgitation. Both possibilities must be excluded by careful questioning and dietary analysis (see also case 40). The appearance of the wear facets suggests erosion as the major cause. Although the teeth interdigitate on incisal enamel, the dentine has been lost from an area which is not in contact with the opposing teeth.
Attrition	Attrition is usually caused by occlusal wear and a minor degree is normal. Bruxism and other parafunctional habits may have caused increased attrition. There is no evidence of masticatory muscle tenderness or hypertrophy to suggest that such habits contribute.
Abrasion	Abrasion of the teeth is wear by an external agent and is seen when a coarse diet is eaten, as in developing countries, or as a result of toothbrush abrasion. There is nothing to suggest an unusual diet in this case, though the possibility should be excluded by questioning. The pattern is not consistent with a primarily abrasive process.

INVESTIGATIONS

■ *What investigations would you perform? Why?*

Dietary analysis is required to determine whether there is excessive dietary acid and to identify the sources of sugars responsible for the caries in several teeth.

Radiographic assessment by means of either a panoramic tomograph or full mouth periapical films is necessary. In view of the fact that the patient has not attended a dentist for a decade, the panoramic tomograph would provide a useful survey of both teeth and edentulous ridges. Periapical films of all standing teeth are a reasonable alternative in this case because the missing teeth reduce the number of films and radiation dose required. A periapical film of the lower left second premolar is required to assess the feasibility of root canal treatment and obtaining films of the other discoloured teeth would be prudent despite their apparent vitality. Periapical films taken with a paralleling technique would allow accurate assessment of bone levels.

Upper and lower study models are required to assess the treatment options for the short clinical crowns and to design a new denture. When restoring extensively worn teeth the models should be mounted in the retruded contact position on either a fully- or semi-adjustable articulator. Obtaining an accurate occlusal record is particularly important in this case because the patient has a habitual forward mandibular posture. Only the retruded contact position is reproducible and only models mounted to this occlusal record can be used to analyse this patient's adapted intercuspal position. The study models can also be used to produce a diagnostic wax-up which is mounted onto the articulator so that it is possible to assess how much the vertical dimension needs increasing to accommodate the crowns. The diagnostic wax-up can be duplicated in stone and a soft vacuum-formed splint (or silicone matrix) formed around it and used to make the provisional crowns.

Assessment of vertical dimension. Most dentate patients will accept the increased vertical dimension needed to create sufficient space for crowns. This would not be so for a mucosa-borne denture, which would probably fail. Although the precise mechanisms are not understood, it is believed that the pain fibres in the periodontal ligament prevent overloading.

DIAGNOSIS

Dietary analysis reveals a moderate sucrose intake as snacks and a moderate citrus fruit and fruit juice component in the diet. The patient is suffering from tooth loss caused primarily by erosion with a secondary element of attrition. The extent of the tooth wear may indicate an element of asymptomatic regurgitation but the patient declined investigation.

TREATMENT PLANNING

■ *What is the main problem in providing crowns for these teeth?*

The short clinical crowns. Further reduction in crown length would be required to create space for the artificial crowns and this would leave short, unretentive preparations.

■ *What two basic treatment philosophies could be used to restore the dentition? What are their advantages and disadvantages and which should be chosen in this case?*

The two basic choices are either to accept short anterior crowns and make a denture to the existing intercuspal position and vertical dimension (the conformative approach) or to restore the teeth in the retruded-contact position (the reorganized approach).

Approach	Advantages and disadvantages
Conformative	The new restorations are placed conforming to the existing occlusal vertical dimension and intercuspal position. This means that the restorations are easier to make and the patient needs to make minimal adaptation to them. The height of the tooth must be reduced further to produce occlusal clearance and this may expose the pulp. The conformative approach is usually the more convenient method for single crowns or simple bridges.
Reorganized	This is required when the vertical dimension or intercuspal position must be altered significantly or when multiple units are needed. In cases of tooth wear, the vertical dimension often needs to be increased and a new occlusal relationship defined to correct the mandibular posture and articulate the crowns. The retruded-contact position is chosen because it is reproducible and can act as the new intercuspal position.

■ *Which approach is necessary in this case and how would you manage the vertical dimension?*

In this case a reorganized approach should be adopted. This is because the crowns of the unrestored teeth are very short. To crown these teeth the natural crown would need to be reduced in height to provide occlusal clearance and this would result in even shorter unretentive preparations. It is therefore necessary to gain space for the new tooth height.

■ *How might this problem be overcome?*

Surgical crown lengthening with alveolar bone remodelling can be used to overcome this problem. The gingival margin is repositioned apically to create a longer tooth, shown in Figure 41.2, which can be prepared for a crown in the conventional manner, shown in Figure 41.3. Crown lengthening does not alter the occlusal vertical dimension because the additional crown length needed for preparation is obtained by exposing the root. Surgical crown lengthening is preferable to electrosurgery which merely alters the gingival contour.

The alternative is to accept the height of the teeth and the gingival contour and create vertical space by adding to the incisal height of the artificial crowns.

In this case the teeth are so short that a combination of both techniques is required.

■ *How is surgical crown lengthening achieved?*

Flaps are raised buccally and palatally and crestal bone is removed with a bur. Both the height of the bone and its width must be adapted, remodelling the alveolar contour so that the soft tissues will return to their new apical position but be able to retain the normal shape of the gingival margin. Bone is removed palatally and buccally. The amount removed must be judged so that sufficient crown length is produced to allow a retentive preparation but support from the root is not compromised. The optimum distance from the crest of the alveolar bone to the gingival margin is 3–4 mm. Sufficient bone must be removed to preserve this distance or the gingival tissues will regrow to their original position.

■ *What are the disadvantages of crown lengthening?*

- Crown lengthening results in the crown margins lying on the root surfaces of the teeth. The cross-sectional area of the root is smaller than the crown so that the preparation is rather tall and narrow (and therefore weak) and the final restoration is more triangular in shape (as in the provisional restorations in Figure 41.3).
- Some patients develop significant sensitivity from the exposed dentine.
- Part of the periodontium is removed. The support of teeth with short roots may be compromised as a result.
- The procedure is uncomfortable for the patient and time is needed for healing and for the new gingival contour to stabilize.

■ *Are there any alternatives to crown lengthening?*

An alternative approach to surgical crown lengthening would be to accept the clinical crown height but gain additional retention by placing a post in the root canal. However, elective root treatment should be avoided whenever possible in cases of tooth wear. This is especially so when there is a significant element of attrition, for instance from a parafunctional habit. The additional occlusal loading may result in decementation of the post or fracture of the root.

Secondary dentine formation below the wear may also complicate root treatment by causing sclerosis of the canal.

■ *The patient clearly dislikes his acrylic partial denture. Will restoration require a replacement?*

Ideally, yes. When the anterior teeth are restored the patient will need sufficient occlusal table posteriorly to masticate effectively.

In the short term an upper partial denture is required, preferably a tooth-supported chrome–cobalt denture. In the longer term other options such as an implant-retained bridge might be considered. However, such complex treatment should not be provided until caries activity has been controlled.

TREATMENT

In this case crown-lengthening surgery was performed on all upper and lower teeth and the vertical dimension was increased to provide additional space for the new crowns. The effect of crown lengthening is shown in Figure 41.2 and the provisonal restorations in Figure 41.3.

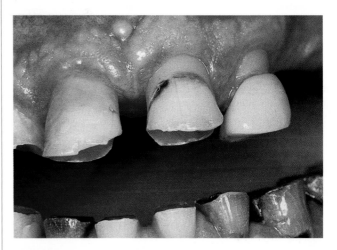

Fig. 41.2 The upper anterior teeth following surgical crown lengthening.

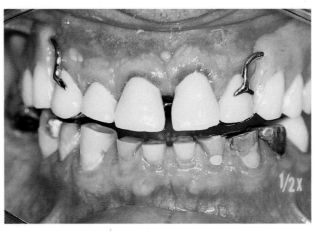

Fig. 41.3 Provisional restorations after crown lengthening.

Table 41.1 Stages of treatment plan

Stage	Reason
Diagnostic wax-up	To show the patient the eventual shape and relationships of the planned crowns. It can also be used to produce the provisional restorations.
Crown-lengthening surgery in upper arch	To gain length for retention. Usually, the upper arch is treated first because it is technically easier. In addition the upper provisional crowns establish the new anterior guidance which can be copied in the definitive restorations once the patient is comfortable.
Healing period	The time delay between the periodontal surgery and placement of provisional crowns should be in the order of a few weeks as there is some evidence that the tissues can heal back towards their original position. Definitive crowns can be made once gingival contour is stable, around 3–4 months post surgery.
Provisional restorations, upper arch	These are made shortly after the crown lengthening and the anterior guidance is adjusted so that the patient is comfortable. The restorations should be worn for at least a few weeks to assess the patient's compliance (Figure 41.3).
New denture and definitive upper restoration	The new crowns are made first and then the denture around them. Some clinicians will make the crowns, try them in and recement the provisional restoration. This allows the denture to be constructed to fit the final crowns in the laboratory. Others prefer to cement the new crowns in place and take a new impression to construct the denture.
Assessment period	Allows time for the patient to decide whether they wish to have the lower arch restored.
Lower arch crown lengthening and new crowns	The same process is used in the lower arch once the surgical procedure is completed. It is unlikely that the patient needs lower teeth posterior to the second premolars.

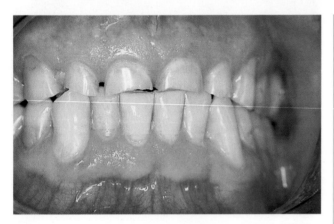

Fig. 41.4 Another patient with marked upper anterior tooth wear.

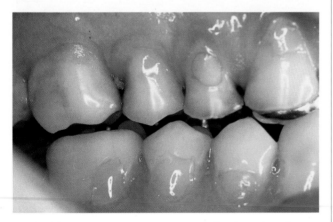

Fig. 41.5 Posterior teeth immediately after insertion of an anterior bite plane.

■ *How should the stages of treatment be organized into a treatment plan culminating in the permanent restoration? Why is each stage required?*

See Table 41.1.

■ *How would your treatment differ for the patient shown in Figure 41.4 who has a complete dentition?*

When more teeth are present the extra vertical space needed to make the crowns can be created orthodontically. An anterior bite plane (Dahl appliance) is cemented to the teeth with a relatively weak cement such as a glass ionomer. This allows the posterior teeth to overerupt and also intrudes the anterior teeth so that tooth movement rather than tooth reduction provides the crown length necessary for retentive crown preparations. The appliance is worn for about 3–6 months, depending on the rate of eruption. The patient's appliance is shown in Figure 41.5 holding the posterior teeth apart at the start of treatment.

CASE

42 A case of toothache

Summary of problem
A 36-year-old Nigerian lady presents in your practice for the first time, complaining of toothache.

HISTORY

Complaint
She complains of toothache associated with her lower left teeth and points somewhat imprecisely to the lower left quadrant.

History of complaint
The patient has been aware of intermittent pain at this site for several months. Initially the pain was short-lived and brought on by hot and cold drinks but in the last few days the discomfort has become progressively worse. She is now suffering a fairly constant and very painful toothache which is no longer closely related to hot and cold stimuli.

Medical history
She is otherwise fit and well and no positive findings are revealed by the medical history.

EXAMINATION

Extraoral examination
She is a fit and well-looking African lady. The submandibular lymph nodes are not palpable. There is no detectable soft tissue swelling and the temporomandibular joints appear normal.

Intraoral examination
The lower left second premolar and first and second permanent molars are heavily restored. There is only a small restoration in the first premolar. Several other teeth contain smaller restorations. The surrounding oral mucosa appears normal and there is no bony enlargement or swelling. No tenderness is elicited on palpation of the lingual or buccal sulcus adjacent to the teeth and the contour of the tissues here is normal.

■ *How do you interpret the history and examination so far?*

The clear history of toothache (which is normally correctly identified by patients) and the large restorations suggest that one or more teeth may be the cause of the pain, probably as a result of caries or complications of restoration. The pain is poorly localized, severe, feels like toothache and has been exacerbated by hot and cold, almost certainly indicating pulpitis. The recent onset of pain unrelated to hot and cold suggests late or irreversible pulpitis but that the causative pulp remains partially vital. The history does not suggest spread of infection or inflammation to the periodontal ligament, which is normally associated with pain on biting and accurate localization of the causative tooth by the patient.

■ *What simple additional examinations would you perform and why?*

All the teeth in the lower left quadrant distal to, and including, the canine should be percussed. The same teeth should be tested for vitality, together with their equivalent lower right teeth for comparison (provided there are no clinical features such as caries or restorations suggesting that these also have compromised vitality).

When this is done, it is found that no teeth are particularly tender to percussion. Both the second premolar and first molar may be slightly tender (the patient is unclear) but neither gives a dull percussive note. The second premolar is vital but the first molar is hypersensitive, both by electric pulp testing and application of a cold stimulus (ethyl chloride).

INVESTIGATIONS

■ *What investigation would you now undertake and why?*

An intraoral periapical radiograph of the lower left premolars and first molar should be taken. The examination so far indicates that the first molar is the most likely cause of the pain. However, the patient is vague as to whether the second premolar is tender to percussion and it contains a large restoration. There may be two causes for the pain. A radiograph cannot provide direct evidence of vitality.

However it will give information on possible causes of loss of vitality, particularly caries and inadequate restorations, as well as revealing previous attempted root canal treatment and periapical granuloma or infection (provided there has been sufficient time for apical bone loss to develop). A radiograph will also be required in the event that either extraction or root canal treatment is necessary.

■ *The periapical radiograph is shown in Figure 42.1. What do you see?*

The periapical radiograph shows:
• A minimal restoration in the first premolar root.

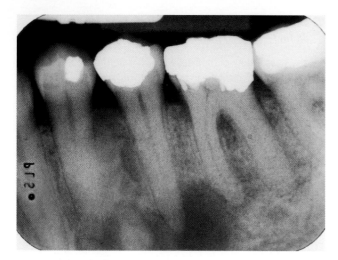

Fig. 42.1 Periapical of both lower premolars and first molar.

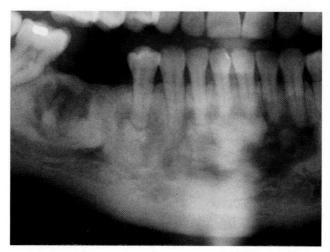

Fig. 42.2 Section from the dental panoramic tomograph.

- Large restorations in the second premolar and first and second molars.
- No radiographic evidence of dental caries.
- Early bifurcation bone loss associated with the first molar.
- A radiolucent area centred on the apex of second premolar which appears to extend to involve the mesial root of the first molar.
- Loss of lamina dura around the apex of the root of the second premolar and the first molar mesial root.
- An irregular but relatively well defined radiopaque zone distal to the first premolar root.

■ *What would you do next and why?*

Further radiographic views are required. The radiograph has not aided diagnosis of the dental pain as no unsuspected cause for the pulpitis has been identified. However it has revealed an apical radiolucency on the second premolar and first molar which is not compatible with an uncomplicated periapical granuloma, infection or cyst. The presence of an apical radiolucency on the second premolar is also incompatible with the history and examination which indicate that this tooth is vital.

The presence of both radiopacity and radiolucency require consideration of a wider differential diagnosis which would include fibro-cemento-osseous lesions, odontogenic tumours and a variety of bone disorders. The margins of the radiolucent lesion are not visible in the film and need to be defined before a more accurate differential diagnosis can be proposed. Because some fibro-cemento-osseous lesions may be bilateral, appropriate views would be a dental panoramic tomograph or right and left oblique laterals. These will also allow all the teeth and their supporting structures to be assessed because the patient is being seen in the practice for the first time. Bitewings to assess caries would also be appropriate in a new patient with several heavily restored teeth if there is clinical suspicion of caries.

■ *Part of the dental panoramic tomograph is shown in Figure 42.2. What do you see?*

The additional radiograph shows several features including:
- The lower right second premolar and first molar are absent, presumed extracted.

- A small occlusal restoration in the lower left second molar which has tipped slightly mesially.
- An extensive lesion of mixed radiodensity involving the central body of the mandible from the mesial root of the second molar across the midline to join that shown previously in the left.
- The lesion appears to be composed of several radiolucencies often with a central opacity centred on the root apices.
- There is little or no expansion of the bone despite the extensive lesion.
- The lesion has not displaced teeth or inferior dental nerve canal.
- There are no lesions in the maxilla (not seen in figure).

DIAGNOSIS

■ *What are the causes of a mixed radiolucency such as this in the jaws?*

- Cemento-osseous dysplasias
  —periapical
  —focal
  —florid
- Chronic osteomyelitis
- Paget's disease of bone
- Fibrous dysplasia
- Metastatic malignancy.

■ *What is the most likely diagnosis? Explain why.*

One of the cemento-osseous dysplasias is the cause of the patient's jaw lesions. The diagnosis may be made on the radiographic appearances alone. No other condition produces multiple lesions centred on the apices of the teeth, each with a central radiopacity and a variable and poorly defined radiolucent rim. As disease progresses this pattern may become less distinct, but it is clearly visible in several of this patient's lesions. This patient has the florid form of the disease in which one or more quadrants are affected. The periapical form affects a few teeth, usually the lower incisors, and the focal form gives rise to one large lesion but all are part of a spectrum of disease severity. The diagnosis is supported by the patient's race, these conditions being more prevalent in those of negroid or mongoloid racial stock. The lesion(s) are normally asymptomatic.

■ *What diagnoses have you excluded? Explain why.*

Chronic osteomyelitis produces a patchy mixed radiolucency but would give symptoms of dull boring central bone pain quite distinct from those reported. Sinuses or other signs of infection would probably be present. However, this diagnosis should not be completely excluded without a further consideration, because the sclerotic bone of fibro-cemento-osseous lesions such as florid cemento-osseous dysplasia is prone to infection, particularly dental infection, and in the past the condition was thought to be a form of osteomyelitis. A biopsy to confirm the presumed diagnosis is contraindicated because of the risk of osteomyelitis.

Paget's disease of bone may be confidently excluded because it never affects the mandible without producing obvious lesions, signs and symptoms in other bones. If this were Paget's disease the maxilla would be affected. Paget's disease affects predominantly elderly Caucasians.

Fibrous dysplasia might be considered as a cause of patchy and poorly defined radiolucency but presents with expansion of the jaw, usually the maxilla, during the first or second decade.

Metastatic malignancy might also be considered as a further cause. Most cancers cause purely radiolucent lesions but some, notably prostate and breast, may cause bony sclerosis and radiopacity. However the site is usually at the angle of the mandible, and the radiological appearances are sufficiently characteristic of florid cemento-osseous dysplasia to exclude this sinister diagnosis.

■ *How might you confirm the diagnosis without biopsy?*

Any previous radiographs should be reviewed to determine whether the lesion has been present and slowly progressing for several years. This would confirm the diagnosis. A previous dental practitioner was contacted and provided the radiograph seen in Figure 42.3 which had been taken 11 years previously.

The radiograph shows the lower left quadrant. The lower left second premolar and first molar contain smaller restorations than at present and there is probable caries in the second premolar. However the first premolar appears to contain the same restoration as at present, and at its apex there is a lesion typical of early cemento-osseous dysplasia comprising a radiolucency with a central opacity at the root apex. This early stage of the lesion provides conclusive evidence for the proposed diagnosis.

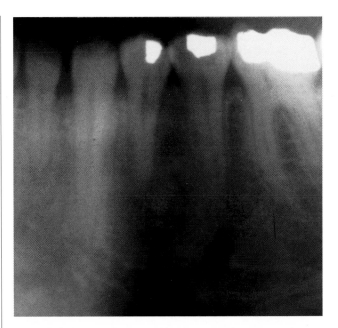

Fig. 42.3 Section from the dental panoramic tomograph taken 11 years previously.

■ *What would you do about the patient's pain?*

The causative tooth must be identified. Vitality must be accurately established and the most effective way to do this is to perform a 'test cavity' in the first molar without local anaesthetic. When this was done the tooth was found to be non-vital and the second premolar was found to be vital. The first molar requires root treatment or extraction. The apical radiolucency on the second premolar is an early radiolucent lesion of cemento-osseous dysplasia and this was confirmed some years later when radiographs revealed that the lesion had developed a zone of radiopacity centrally.

■ *Does florid cemento-osseous dysplasia have any significant complications?*

Yes. Precautions must be taken to ensure that the patient does not develop osteomyelitis in the sclerotic bone of the mandible. A preventive regime for caries and periodontal disease must be instituted to reduce the chances of future dental infection. The periodontal condition of the first molar is poor and extraction would be the preferred option. Other nonvital teeth should also be extracted if there are reasons to suspect that root canal treatment may not be successful. Antibiotics should be prescribed during the healing period for all extractions involving affected bone. Any surgery in the mandible should be similarly covered and would be best performed in hospital rather than general practice unless the practitioner has appropriate experience.

A child with a swollen face

Summary

A 5-year-old boy has painless bilateral facial swellings. Identify the cause and recommend treatment.

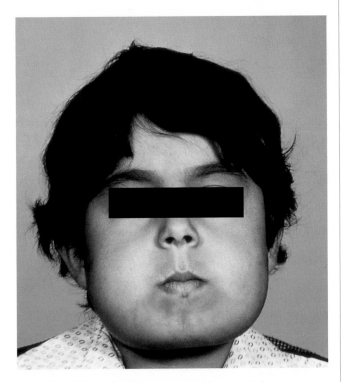

Fig. 43.1 The patient's appearance at presentation.

HISTORY

Complaint

The patient is brought by his parents who have noticed that his face has become fat. They are concerned about his appearance and say that he is being teased and bullied at school.

History of complaint

His parents say that the patient has had a chubby face since he was a toddler but that the swelling has become more noticeable over the last 2 years. He is in no pain.

Medical history

He is otherwise fit and well, has had all recommended immunizations and amongst the childhood illnesses has suffered only chicken pox. His medical practitioner has given him a general examination and found no systemic illness but has referred him to you for a further opinion.

EXAMINATION

Extraoral examination

The appearance of the child is shown in Figure 43.1. He appears healthy but has obvious bilateral enlargement of the side of the face. The temporo-mandibular joints appear normal on palpation. Some upper deep cervical lymph nodes are palpable bilaterally. They are only slightly enlarged, not tender and are freely mobile.

■ *On the basis of what you know, what types of lesion would you consider?*

From this view alone it is difficult to tell whether the swelling originates in the salivary glands, mandible or soft tissues. Each site would have different possible causes:

Condition	Possible causes
Salivary gland enlargement	Rare in children. HIV salivary cystic disease is seen in HIV infection but there is nothing else to suggest HIV infection. Mumps can be excluded. Mumps is acute and, in addition, the child would have had mumps vaccine with the rest of the routine childhood vaccinations.
Enlargement of the mandible	A few rare inherited disorders of bone could cause bilateral expansion of the ramus.
A developmental syndrome	Many syndromes have craniofacial signs and this is a possibility which should be borne in mind. There appear to be no associated features.

Intraoral examination

Intraoral examination reveals a minimally restored dentition and healthy oral mucosa. Palpation of the mandibular rami shows that they are the source of the enlargement. There is obvious rounded swelling of the posterior body and ramus of the mandible. The lower right second deciduous molar is missing.

INVESTIGATIONS

■ *A radiograph is obviously required. Which view(s) would you choose?*

A dental panoramic tomograph is the investigation of choice as an initial view. The whole of the swellings will be visible and the left and right can be easily compared. A posterior–anterior view of the jaws would also be useful, providing a second view at right angles to the ramus in the panoramic view. It would allow mediolateral expansion to be assessed.

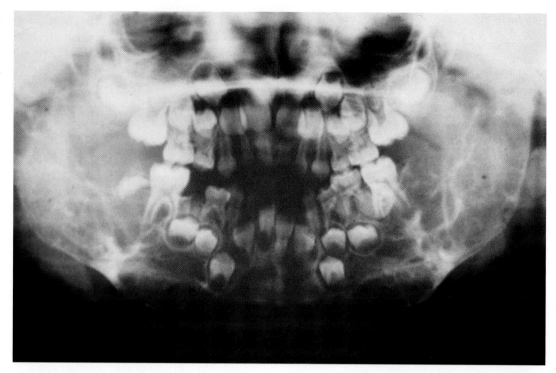

Fig. 43.2 Dental panoramic tomograph.

■ *The radiographic appearance is shown in Figure 43.2. What are the radiographic features of the lesions?*

See Table 43.1

Table 43.1 Radiographic features

Site	Bilaterally in the posterior body, angle and ascending rami of the mandible.
Size	Relatively large, about 5 × 8 cm.
Shape	Lesions on both sides are multilocular.
Type of outline/edge	Smooth, well defined and well corticated.
Relative radiodensity	Radiolucent with internal radiopaque septa producing a multilocular appearance. There are no dense radiopaque inclusions.
Effects on adjacent structures	Gross displacement of the developing permanent second molars. The lower right second deciduous molar has been lost, presumably by exfoliation. There has been extensive expansion of the height of the body of the mandible. The condyles are not affected.

DIFFERENTIAL DIAGNOSIS

■ *Give a differential diagnosis. Explain which is the most likely cause and why.*

Only a very short differential diagnosis is possible for this case.

Diagnosis	Similarity to present case
Cherubism	Causes bilateral radiolucencies in the mandibular rami and maxilla. Enlargement starts in children before the age of 5 years. The lesions appear multilocular and radiolucent and disrupt the dentition. The radiographic and facial appearances in this case are characteristic.
Other possible causes	There are a few very rare bone diseases and syndromes which may need to be considered if the most likely diagnosis of cherubism cannot be confirmed. Almost all other causes have prominent signs elsewhere in the body and none have been noted in this case.

■ *What further questions might help confirm your diagnosis?*

Did either parent have a similar problem? Cherubism is inherited in an autosomal dominant fashion. It would be expected that one parent would be similarly affected. Females are often less severely affected and cases may appear to be sporadic. Radiographs of both parents may reveal healed lesions and this would aid diagnosis.

Are any brothers or sisters affected? For similar reasons, siblings would be expected to show similar signs.

How was the lower second deciduous molar lost? Cherubism may cause exfoliation of teeth.

■ *Would any further radiographs help confirm the diagnosis?*

More detailed radiographic examination with intraoral films would be helpful for the following reasons.
- To demonstrate involvement of the maxilla. More severely affected patients usually have smaller lesions in the maxilla, usually centred on the tuberosity but sometimes extending to distort the orbit. These can easily be missed on extraoral films but, if present, confirm the diagnosis.
- To identify displacement or destruction of teeth. As noted above, cherubism often destroys tooth germs and displaces teeth.

■ *Is a biopsy required?*

In a classical case of cherubism, the diagnosis may be made with certainty on the basis of family history, clinical and radiographic features. In a new case such as this, or if there were no family history, it would be prudent to confirm that the lesions are histologically compatible with cherubism.

■ *A biopsy specimen was removed from the expanded alveolar ridge. The histological appearances are shown in Figure 43.3. What do you see?*

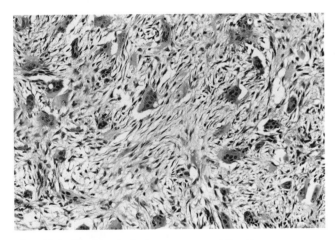

Fig. 43.3 The histological appearance of the biopsy specimen.

The lesion is composed of cellular fibrous tissue which appears loose and oedematous with spaces rather than dense collagen between the cells. Scattered in the fibrous tissue are multinucleate giant cells. These are relatively small giant cells and have only 4–8 nuclei each.

■ *How do you interpret these appearances? Are they consistent with cherubism?*

Lesions with many giant cells fall into two broad categories, those with granulomas, such as tuberculosis, sarcoidosis and foreign body reactions, and the *giant-cell lesions*. No granulomas are present and these appearances indicate a giant-cell lesion, the causes of which are:
- central giant-cell granuloma
- brown tumour of hyperparathyroidism
- aneurysmal bone cyst
- cherubism.

These conditions cannot be distinguished from one another on histological grounds alone. However, the only one which matches the clinical and radiographic findings is cherubism.

DIAGNOSIS

Taken together, the evidence supports a diagnosis of cherubism and this is a typical case.

TREATMENT

■ *What treatment would you recommend? What other advice would you give to the parents?*

No treatment is required though the parents and child may need reassurance. The parents can be told that lesions of cherubism usually grow fastest before the age of 5. Although there will be further growth during the next few years, the lesions will stop growing spontaneously and start to regress around the age of puberty. The swelling should have completely resolved by the age of 25 and only radiographic changes will remain into the fourth decade.

Surgical intervention is not usually necessary but may be performed for cosmetic reasons if lesions resolve slowly. Some teeth will be lost through the disease process. The parents should also be warned that future children and siblings are likely to be affected. Genetic counselling would be appropriate.

Index